Dr Dilys Davies is a clinical psychologist and qualified psychotherapist who specializes in sleep difficulties. She is Secretary of the psychotherapy section of the British Psychological Society, an advisor to the World Health Organization on the treatment of insomnia.

THE ELEMENT GUIDE SERIES

The *Element Guide* series addresses important
psychological and emotional issues in a clear,
authoritative and straightforward manner. The
series is designed for all people who deal with these
issues as everyday challenges. Each book explores
the background, possible causes and symptoms
where appropriate, and presents a comprehensive
approach to coping with the situation. Each book
also includes advice on self-help, as well as where –
and when – to turn for qualified help. The books are
objective and accessible, and lead the reader to a
point where they can make informed decisions
about where to go next.

Titles in the Element Guide series

INSOMNIA

Your Questions Answered

Dr Dilys Davies

ELEMENT

Shaftesbury, Dorset • Boston, Massachusetts
Melbourne, Victoria

© Element Books Limited 1999
Text © Dr Dilys Davies 1999

First published in the UK in 1999 by
Element Books Limited
Shaftesbury, Dorset SP7 8BP

Published in the USA in 1999 by
Element Books, Inc.
160 North Washington Street
Boston, MA 02114

Published in Australia in 1999 by
Element Books and distributed by
Penguin Australia Limited
487 Maroondah Highway, Ringwood, Victoria 3134

Cover illustration by Lesley Ann Hutchins
Cover design by The Bridgewater Book Company
Design by Roger Lightfoot
Typeset by WestKey Limited, Falmouth, Cornwall
Printed and bound in Great Britain by
Biddles Ltd, Guildford & King's Lynn

British Library Cataloguing in Publication
data available

Library of Congress Cataloging in Publication
data available

ISBN 1 86204 296 9

Note from the Publisher
Any information given in any book in the *Element Guide* series is not
intended to be taken as a replacement for medical advice. Any person
with a condition requiring medical attention should consult a qualified
medical practitioner or suitable therapist.

Contents

This book is dedicated to J. Richard Marshall (1945–1995), my fellow owl, and to my mother, Elisabeth Mary Davies, one of life's larks.

Acknowledgements

I am grateful to Dr Philip McLean for his academic advice and contributions. My gratitude also goes to Dr Rachel Daley and Dr Ashwin Patkar for their help. I would like to thank Martin Doherty, Jane and Gordon Garrick, Fiona McLean, Norma Maple, Andrea McGlashan and Rowena Jackson for their unfailing encouragement. Also I would like to thank Rhodri Wilkins and Siân Thomas who facilitated the process of writing this book. My thanks go to my editor Grace Cheetham for her support and patience and her contribution in structuring this book. Lastly a special thank-you goes to the many patients with whom I worked in the sleep clinic whose stories and experiences taught me about insomnia.

Introduction

Sleep is such a normal natural part of our lives that when we sleep well we take it for granted and barely think about how we sleep or why it seems such an essential part of living.

However, for many people a good, uninterrupted night's sleep is hard to come by. Most of us have had the odd sleepless night, but after a night or so our usual sleep pattern is restored. However, if sleeplessness continues either through not being able to go off to sleep, waking on and off during the night, with difficulty in dropping off again, or waking early in the morning, we feel tired and less able physically and mentally to cope with the next day's events. Pretty soon we feel physically exhausted and emotionally drained. This is what is called insomnia, and it is one of the most common health problems, affecting up to a third of the population. However, these days there is a great deal that most people suffering from insomnia can do for themselves. This book outlines the different types of insomnia and their possible causes, and shows you how to assess your own sleep pattern, explore the nature of your sleep problems and start making changes to bring about better sleep.

There are many causes for poor sleep. Many sleeping problems are brought about by people basing their ideas about sleep on myths and remedies which actually make the condition worse. For example, the notion that eight hours' sleep a night is essential for our well-being is a myth. Everyone has a different sleep pattern – some people need as little as three hours' sleep while others need as long as ten or more hours a night. The amount of sleep we need varies through our lives and also depends on the sort of things we do and how we do them during the day. What is important is that you find out what the right amount of sleep is for you.

For most of us, sleeping difficulties often result because we have not developed a regular sleep pattern or our usual pattern has been disrupted in some way. This can happen for many reasons, such as in a crisis when it is common for people to react by losing sleep. If sleeplessness continues for too long after the upsetting event our bodies get used to this new tendency and it becomes difficult to correct. Then the sleep problem becomes a habit which is hard to break. This book outlines techniques and strategies that will help you identify and correct poor sleep habits.

Whatever the cause of your insomnia, sleeplessness is often a symptom of some kind of problem in your daytime life. It is a sign that something in your life is out of balance. Problems may be emotional, physical or environmental or often some combination of these. They may be to do with stresses in your working life or lack of work, or because you are dissatisfied, unhappy or depressed for some reason. Poor sleep can then be made even worse by, for example, poor nutritional habits. These are daytime problems that need to be dealt with during the day.

The Element Guide: Insomnia shows how we can learn to understand more about ourselves. It shows how to identify what those patterns are, the way they came about and what kind of feelings, thoughts and attitudes keep them going. Once you know what they are and understand them you can plan to change the old patterns that are not working for you any more and explore new ways. This book helps you to begin to look at ways to sleep better at night by helping you to take a good look at how you go about your daytime activities and assisting you to balance your lifestyle.

Many people feel so desperate at not having enough sleep that they resort to using large amounts of alcohol, tranquillizers and sleeping pills to get what little rest they can. Although the occasional sleeping pill taken on your doctor's advice will not harm you and can help restore a better sleep pattern, these days doctors are much less inclined to prescribe pills for insomnia because they, as well as patients, are concerned about the side-effects. Nightly use of them is ineffective after a few weeks and long-term use can lead to physical and/or psychological addiction. In this book you will also find safer alternatives to sleeping pills, such as natural therapies, including homeopathy and herbalism which many people find helpful in restoring natural sleep.

As soon as you decide to tackle insomnia and work on a plan of action you will not only improve your sleep pattern, you will also be on the way to taking action towards a more satisfactory daytime life and a positive future.

CHAPTER 1

Sleep and Insomnia

WHAT IS SLEEP?

There are many beliefs about what constitutes 'normal', 'natural' or 'good' sleep. However, most of these beliefs have been influenced by culture and history rather than scientifically based biological facts. In fact, much of the folklore about sleep is based on the experience of people whose sleep–wake pattern was determined by the daily rhythm of light and darkness. Until the beginning of the 20th century people's sleep pattern depended on how much light there was during the day. As there was no electricity most people went to bed as daylight faded and got up shortly before dawn. This gave rise to a sleep pattern of about eight to twelve hours a night.

During pre-industrial times, when daily living patterns tended to follow the seasons of the year, the sleep time of most people varied as the days lengthened and shortened with the seasons. The dark winter months with long nights were spent mostly indoors – a pattern which was not very different from the hibernating habits of many mammals. This natural rhythm of life was changed during the second half of the 19th century by the Industrial Revolution. The whole structure of newly industrialized societies was

based on a new time–work ethic: time itself had to be organized in order to meet the demands of industry. With the
introduction of technology the rhythm of nature was
replaced by the rhythm of machines.

There were two major implications to this. First, time
became regimented as machines were turned on or off at a
set time. Second, work was costed in terms of time spent
working, so that time became equated with money. People
were now required to work the hours set by the machine
and its owners instead of following the traditional ways of
watching and waiting and adapting to the needs of nature.
The whole rhythm of life changed, including the pace at
which people worked, the rest periods they took, how
much time they had to themselves and how much and
when they could sleep. When electric light came along at
the beginning of the 20th century, even the hours of darkness could now be used for the needs of production. In this
way standard work times evolved to meet the demands of
industrialization.

As a result our current sleep patterns and ideas about
sleep are very new in evolutionary terms, and very artificial compared with other living creatures. We must therefore be careful when we talk about the 'facts' of normal
sleep and how we understand sleep problems. It is very
easy to forget about the influence technology has had on
the organization of our modern way of life. What we
describe as 'normal' or 'natural' may not be 'normal' or
'natural' at all, but simply a reflection of the way that we
now organize our lives.

WHY DO WE NEED TO SLEEP?

Sleep takes up about a third of our lives. It is part of our
natural daily rhythm, and our own experience tells us that
sleep gives us essential rest, without which we feel tired
and irritable and don't function as well as we'd like the
next day. However, there is still a great deal that we don't

know about how and why we sleep. Research studies carried out in universities and sleep laboratories show that we need less sleep than we think we need and having less sleep does not cause us any harm. The two main functions of sleep are rest and growth.

Rest

When we are asleep parts of our brain and body used for complicated activity during the day are resting. During sleep the heart and lungs rest, the heart rate is reduced and breathing is slow and deep. Blood pressure, pulse rate and body temperature fall, the muscles relax and the body's metabolic rate is reduced. According to Professor Jim Horne, sleep is needed mainly to rest the brain.

Growth

A great deal of activity which is different from the daytime pattern is carried out during sleep. Many important hormones are released, such as those to do with growth and recuperation. The cells of our bodies grow and are repaired during the night. However, some researchers, such as Professor Jim Horne, suggest that for this to happen periods of relaxing or 'relaxed wakefulness' can be as effective as sleep.

DIFFERENCES IN PEOPLE'S SLEEP CYCLES

The body clock: circadian rhythms

As we saw earlier, our sleep–wake rhythms are naturally linked to the cycle of the sun's rising and setting. The way our bodies work is governed by a biological inner clock known as the 'circadian rhythm' (from the Latin *circa diem*, meaning 'about a day'). For example, it regulates the times when various organs become more or less active and when the production of various hormones peaks and tails off. The length of the circadian day is normally between 24 and 25 hours. However, there are differences between people in their sleep cycles.

Researchers studying our internal rhythms have put people in isolated situations, away from natural light and all other external clues as to the passage of time. Their findings show that although most people usually fall into a regular 'day' of about 25 hours, some have a longer natural 'day' period and adopt a cycle of 26 or 27 hours. Thus some people have difficulty keeping to a regular 24-hour cycle as their internal clocks are less influenced by the world's 24-hour day.

The circadian rhythm is set to bring on sleep twice a day, mainly at night but also in the early afternoon, which is why many of us feel sleepy after lunch. The siesta, traditional in many hot countries, is declining as business takes on a global nature and air-conditioning is becoming established. Yet it could be much more natural than our own patterns.

The circadian rhythm also varies with age. Babies sleep regularly during the day, at first around three-hourly intervals, tailing off to a morning and an afternoon sleep. By the age of about two and a half they are sleeping in the afternoon only. In the elderly the need for an afternoon sleep usually returns.

Owls and larks

Generally, we tend to fall into two main categories. There are those of us who are best in the morning and see ourselves as 'morning people' and those of us who function best in the evening and view ourselves as 'night people'. In other words, we are what Professor Jim Horne calls either owls or larks. Larks are people who are naturally at their peak in the morning. Owls are most alert and productive later in the day or at night. Numerically, there are more larks than owls.

Larks tend to get up at an early hour and are wide awake within half an hour, geared up for the events of the day. During the day their level of wakefulness sags from time to time. The first of these low spots is about 10.30 in the morning when blood sugars run low, and it is at this time of day that accidents are most common at work or while driving. Society's answer to this is the coffee-break. Another low period comes after lunch and perhaps in the late afternoon when some larks are tempted to nap. They get steadily less alert during the late hours of the day until bedtime when they sleepily go to bed and quickly fall into a deep sleep.

The owl or night person has a very different pattern. They struggle to wake up and battle through the first hour and a half of the day. As the day goes on owls become increasingly more alert in a fluctuating way until evening when they reach their peak. From 11.30pm onwards while the rest of the world goes to bed the lone owl is often left wide awake but with no one to play with. Unlike the larks, the owl typically has difficulty going to sleep and tends to stay in light sleep longer than other people before drifting into deep sleep. Some owls may still be in a relatively deep sleep when the time comes to wake up in the morning and start the day. There is some evidence that owls adjust better to the reversed sleep–wake schedules that are necessary for night-shift work. Perhaps one day we owls will demand a better deal but at present we must keep bravely struggling on and adjust to a society which is organized to suit the majority of people – the larks.

STAGES OF SLEEP

Research on sleep shows there are four stages of sleep. Each stage slips into the next and the whole cycle lasts about 90 minutes. Each stage has a different pattern of brain activity which can be monitored by EEG (electro-encephalogram) recordings in sleep laboratories. (In the waking state our brains usually emit fast beta waves which have a frequency of around 15 cycles per second.)

Stage 1 sleep

This first stage is the lightest and is the shift from wakeful-ness to drowsiness. It is similar to when we relax or rest. Any noise can easily awaken us fully during this stage. As we enter this stage our muscles relax, blood pressure drops, heart rate and digestion slow down. The brain begins to produce hormones such as serotonin and mela-tonin which are associated with sleep and sleepiness, although whether they actually cause sleep is still unclear. During this stage there is an increase in alpha waves, brain waves of 7–14 cycles per second, which are typical of relaxed wakefulness. These alpha waves also occur when people are meditating or are under hypnosis. This stage lasts between one and ten minutes in the normal sleeper although we return to it at intervals during the night. It usually takes up only about 5 per cent of our sleep.

Stage 2 sleep

This second stage starts quite soon after falling asleep. Generally, noise will not disturb us and wake us up although noises which are significant to us – such as hear-ing a child cry or hearing our own name being called out – can wake us up. In this stage there is a mixture of deeper, slower brain waves, typical of drowsiness and light sleep, called theta brain waves (3.5–7.5 cycles per second), and slow delta waves (under 3.5 cycles per second) during which we are, in effect, unconscious. This stage takes up about 45 per cent of our sleep and merges with stage 3 sleep.

Stage 3 sleep

During this third stage on our way to deeper sleep our heart rate slows, our temperature falls and we breathe more slowly. This stage takes up only about 7 per cent of sleep. As delta wave activity increases, we are taken fairly quickly into stage 4 sleep.

Stage 4 sleep

This is the deepest sleep, when delta brain waves predominate. We find it difficult to wake up during this stage. It makes up about 13 per cent of sleep. We stay in stage 4 for quite long periods before slipping back upwards through stages 3, 2 and 1 until we almost wake up. At this point we've actually moved into another kind of sleep called REM sleep.

REM sleep

REM or Rapid Eye Movement sleep is so called because of the rapid eye movements that can be seen under our eyelids during this stage. It is also called 'paradoxical sleep' because although the brain is active the body experiences a kind of paralysis and can't move voluntarily. It is during this stage that we dream, whether we remember doing so or not, although it has now been found that we also dream during deeper stages of sleep. REM sleep happens during stage 1 and lasts for about 10 minutes, although it increases later on during the night. Then we slide down again into the next 90-minute cycle. This time we stay in stage 4 sleep for less time, then come up again to a longer period of up to 20 minutes' REM sleep. During the remaining two or three 90-minute cycles we sleep less deeply and REM sleep increases.

WHAT SORT OF SLEEP DO WE NEED?

It was thought at one time that REM sleep was essential for brain rest and that without it our mental health would suffer. This is now thought not to be the case, although studies carried out in sleep laboratories show that when people are totally deprived of REM sleep for more than three days they start to have waking dreams and begin to hallucinate.

Some researchers such as Professor Jim Horne suggest that possibly too much attention has been paid to the importance of REM sleep. He also suggests that the really essential part of sleep consists of stages 3 and 4, which he calls Slow Wave Sleep (SWS). During these stages the brain is what he calls 'off line' as it is the only time that the brain is totally at rest. SWS occurs mostly during the first three sleep cycles – that is, during the first half of a night's sleep. Studies show that when people are deprived of sleep – for example, by staying up all night – they don't need to catch up with all the sleep they have lost. When they sleep after having lost a night's sleep, they recover all the first deep sleep and some REM sleep, which suggests that this is the sleep that is really essential for us.

Jim Horne concludes that as long as we get our supply of what he calls 'core sleep', consisting of SWS and some REM sleep, the brain will recover from the wear and tear of waking life. The remainder he calls 'optional sleep' which may not be really necessary but fills in the hours after the essential core sleep.

People who naturally need less sleep than average follow the same sleep pattern during the first few hours of sleep as the average person's pattern. They simply cut down on the later non-essential hours of sleep while still getting the essential SWS.

HOW MUCH SLEEP DO WE REALLY NEED?

However bad their sleep pattern, people typically get more sleep than they think they've had, although it's often difficult to convince them of this. Some people try and live by the myth that eight hours' sleep is essential to their well-being, even though they personally may need only five hours' sleep a night. They then wake up convinced they haven't had enough sleep and may lie in bed in the morning restless and miserable as they try to catch up on the sleep they don't, in fact, need. Lying in then makes the problem worse. Similarly, people may try going to bed too early, convinced that if they don't get what they believe to be their full quota of sleep they'll feel dreadful the next day. However, all this does is to set up a pattern of worrying and uncomfortable restlessness which prevents them sleeping as they try even harder to get the sleep they don't really need.

Researchers suggest that around six hours is adequate for our mental health. As discussed earlier in this chapter, any sleep after that comes in the category of 'optional' sleep. What the brain needs is 'core sleep' which predominates during the first sleep cycle. Even if you only sleep for a few hours you'll be getting a period of this important deep sleep together with some REM sleep. Sleep research studies using EEG readings show that some people who feel that they've only slept an hour or two have actually slept for seven hours. Sleep research also shows that people who normally sleep for seven to eight hours can adapt over time to as little as two or three hours' sleep a night without impairing their mental or physical ability. Knowing these facts alone should reassure some insomniacs.

Variations in our sleep needs

It is important to remember that the sleep needs of individuals vary enormously during the course of their lives. For example, some babies naturally need very little sleep while some older people still require a full night's sleep, especially if they remain active and don't nap.

Babies to adolescents

Most small babies sleep about 16–18 hours a day and toddlers still need much more sleep than adults. Children need more while they are growing due to the regeneration of cells during sleep. With adolescence some teenagers will sleep up to 15 hours a night. This is not always due to laziness. However, long sleeping hours are also a symptom of depression which can affect teenagers and is often unrecognized. Our sleep patterns tend to stabilize into our adult patterns at about 16 years of age.

Adults

Research shows that the average young adult sleeps for about seven and a half hours a night. But findings vary. Some surveys show the average to be nearer six and a half hours a night. Generally studies point out that 65 per cent of young adults sleep between 6.5 and 8.5 hours and 95 per cent between 5.5 and 9.5 hours. However, it is important to remember that these figures are just averages and that the amount of sleep needed or taken by people varies a lot. The 'average' 7.5 hours applies to adults between the ages of 16 and 50 years.

Women

Excessive sleepiness in the first three months of pregnancy is normal. Pregnant women also tend to sleep about two more hours a night than usual. In some women the menopause temporarily disrupts sleeping patterns.

Older people

As we get older, night-time sleep becomes lighter and more interrupted with fewer dreams. Also, many older people nap and so need less sleep at night. Including naps, the average sleep for 70-year-olds is about 6 hours in every 24. It's important to realize this since many older people ask for help for their 'sleeping difficulties' when they are, in fact, sleeping quite normally for their age.

How do you know when you have had enough sleep?

You can easily answer this question. Discount the first half-hour after you wake while your metabolism rises to a level of full wakefulness. Then if at full waking you feel refreshed, you've had enough sleep. Studies show that the occasional loss of a night's sleep won't harm you and doesn't have to be made up. People can be kept awake for up to 65 hours with no noticeable effects on the way they function the next day.

SLEEP MYTHS

We can now begin to sense how many myths there are about what constitutes 'normal' or 'natural' sleep. Two of the most popular are the following.

The 'eight-hour' myth

It is difficult to put an exact figure on how much sleep we individually need. Some people need as little as three to four hours while others need up to nine hours or more a night. People's genuine need should not be interpreted as laziness. Most adults sleep for six to eight hours while a few 'drug' themselves with too much sleep.

'Sleeping like a log'

As we have seen, our depth of sleep varies with the stages of sleep. There are periods of very deep sleep called 'orthodox' sleep in which the body is very calm and still, followed by periods of 'paradoxical' sleep which are the high-activity dreaming periods.

SLEEP AND DREAMING

REM sleep, which is associated with dreaming, starts about forty-five minutes after we fall asleep and increases as the night goes on, with most dreaming taking place in the latter part of the night during what is sometimes called 'optional' sleep. During a single night's sleep the average dreaming phase occurs about every 90 minutes so the average sleeper spends about an hour and a half each night in REM sleep, sometimes more.

The amount of dreaming declines with age. Newborn babies spend an enormous amount of time in REM sleep, but whether they are actually dreaming can't be known for certain.

Why do we dream?

There are many different theories about why we dream and the significance that can be attached to our dreams. Psychoanalysts such as Freud and Jung believed that dreams are the road to the unconscious and can show us our hidden feelings and desires. Generally, research psychologists disagree with this view. Some research studies suggest that we dream to re-order stored information and to consolidate memories and learning. Other researchers view dreams as being the result of the brain discarding information, like the 'delete' symbol on a word processor, and that remembering dreams may therefore be bad for us. Yet other researchers suggest that dreams may serve the purpose of being a sort of cinema of the mind, or a way of keeping the brain entertained during lighter stages of sleep.

What seems most likely is that all these theories contain an element of truth. Some dreams are just clearing out rubbish, some are the result of indigestion, while others make us more aware of unresolved problems or suggest answers to them. People have certainly experienced dreams that are emotionally healing or act as a source to creativity. Both poetry and scientific ideas have been inspired by dreams and many people have no doubt about the predictive value of some dreams.

If you're interested in dream content, it can be useful to keep a dream diary. As we can forget dreams very quickly, keep some paper and a pencil by your bed and try to write them down as soon as you wake up. With practice you'll probably find that you remember more of your dreams. Your dreams can symbolize things that are personally meaningful to you. If you're not sure what a dream means, try writing it down first, rather than looking up standard meanings for dream symbols, as sometimes their meaning becomes clearer in the process of writing. As you note down your dreams every night you may begin to notice certain themes coming up which could shed some light on a problem or on your understanding of yourself.

As far as insomnia is concerned, dreams and nightmares are important when they are part of the problem – for example, if they regularly cause you to wake frequently during the night or you awaken in a state of fear. If you have unpleasant recurring dreams, your mind may be trying to draw your attention to something that needs to be dealt with, perhaps a past event that you may have not come to terms with or a present problem like a difficult relationship. In such cases some form of counselling or psychotherapy may be helpful.

WHAT IS INSOMNIA?

Insomnia is one of the most common health complaints, with a third of the population suffering from insomnia at some time or other in their lives. It is defined as a difficulty in initiating and/or maintaining sleep over a period of at least three weeks. Most of us, from time to time, have the odd sleepless night. Usually we can put up with this and after a night or so our usual sleep pattern returns. However, if our sleeping difficulty continues then we feel less able to cope mentally and physically with our daily lives.

Chronic insomnia can last for years, while intermittent insomnia can be triggered by particular anxieties or crises. For example, a common and natural reaction to a crisis is loss of sleep. Although for most people normal sleep returns once the crisis is over, for others sleeplessness can continue long afterwards. By then we've developed poor sleep habits which, like any other habit, once established are difficult to break.

Insomnia can also be a sign that something in our lives is out of balance. This may be emotional, environmental or physical. It may be to do with work or home life, or even general unhappiness.

Conditioned insomnia

Sometimes insomnia can develop into a habit due to what psychologists call 'conditioning'. In such cases, insomnia often starts with an immediate or short-term crisis or emotional upset. During upsetting times people often don't sleep and lying in bed becomes associated with unhappiness and sleeplessness. This association is what is termed 'conditioning'. People whose insomnia is conditioned in this way often sleep very well when they are away from their usual bedroom.

Some conditioned insomnia starts in childhood. For example, people who were sent to bed when they were small for being naughty may associate bed and bedtime with anger and punishment. Some children are sent to bed long before they are really sleepy. They lie awake feeling bored and develop a habit of wakefulness which continues long into adulthood. Others may have been taught by an over-anxious parent that without eight hours' sleep their health would suffer. As a consequence they may suffer from anxiety in later life unless they get their 'eight hours'. This anxiety may in turn keep them awake at night.

Basic types of insomnia

There are three basic types of insomnia. They are:

1 *Difficulty in getting off to sleep*

This is the type of insomnia when we toss and turn for what feels like hours before we can get off to sleep at night.

2 *Intermittent sleep*

This is when we wake up on and off during the night and feel that we never get a good night's sleep.

3 *Early morning wakening*

The third type of insomnia concerns waking early in the morning and not being able to go back to sleep again despite trying.

It is important to remember that the division of insomnia into types is not absolute and any person can suffer a mixture of all three types. Different types of insomnia have traditionally been related to different states of mind. It has been suggested that not being able to get off to sleep at night is a symptom of anxiety while waking early is a sign of depression. However, clinically the picture is often more complicated. While some depressed people cannot get off to sleep, some anxious people fall asleep normally but wake in the early hours. When anxious and depressed, some people sleep more than usual as this may be their way to escape from their problems.

As people's sleep needs vary greatly, insomnia cannot be measured by the number of hours you sleep. Research studies suggest that some insomniacs actually sleep longer than the 'average' person or longer than people who state that they have no difficulties with their sleep. However, if you need ten hours and only sleep for eight, you won't feel as refreshed as the good sleeper who may only need seven hours of sleep.

Insomnia is a subjective state and as such you are the best judge of whether or not you are an insomniac. The main criterion for insomnia is whether as well as experiencing wakefulness during the night you consistently feel that tiredness is affecting your mood and functioning during the next day. For example, if you feel sleepy, tired and irritable throughout the day and your lack of sleep is affecting your memory, concentration and ability to work, you are likely to be suffering from insomnia. Even if you don't sleep for many hours during the night, as long as you feel well and not tired next day you aren't suffering from insomnia. However, worrying unnecessarily about how little sleep you get can be just as stressful as not sleeping and can in itself bring about poor sleep.

If you think you are an insomniac, there are three important things to remember.

1 You may be getting more sleep than you think.
2 As long as you can get some sleep and can relax your body, you won't come to any long-term harm.

3 Your attitude towards your sleep has a lot to do with the quality of the sleep you get.

MEDICAL CONDITIONS ASSOCIATED WITH SLEEP DISORDERS

Insomnia is most frequently related to psychological factors such as emotional stress, attitudes and expectations about sleep, poor sleep habits or even physical or environmental causes. However, there are some specific medical problems associated with sleep disorders. If you're suffering from excessive sleepiness during the day it may be advisable to seek the advice of your family doctor before assuming you're suffering from insomnia. Common medical conditions associated with sleep problems include the following.

Restless legs syndrome

This is a very irritating and uncomfortable syndrome consisting of discomfort in one or both legs and the urge to keep moving them. It keeps you awake even when the rest of you wants to sleep. Its actual cause isn't fully known but it has been suggested that it is connected with poor circulation and/or lack of calcium or other nutrients including vitamin E. In women it may be related to hormone levels. It is often worse when the sufferer is under stress. One strategy is to improve the circulation in your legs by taking a foot bath, alternating hot and cold water, during the evening. Another recommendation is that taking calcium in some form at bedtime can be helpful.

Sleep apnea

This condition, which is increasingly being diagnosed as a problem, is more frequently diagnosed in the USA, possibly because of greater awareness by physicians. Sufferers may be less aware of their sleeping problem than their partners as the most obvious sign is loud, irregular snoring. Sleep apnea occurs in people who have an obstruction at the back of the throat. As the throat relaxes in sleep, their breathing is cut off and the oxygen level in the blood drops. Sufferers don't usually wake fully, but reach a near-waking state in order to breathe again, usually with a loud snort and sometimes with thrashing around. In severe cases this can happen throughout the night. As a result, apnea sufferers never get into the deep stages of sleep and are tired throughout the next day. They can suffer from loss of concentration and memory and are at risk of nodding off during the day – for example, at meetings or while driving. Apnea can also place strain on the heart. The danger is that these symptoms can often be ignored and seen as merely signs of getting older.

Sleep apnea is most commonly found in overweight men who often drink a fair amount of alcohol. Being overweight makes the condition worse by narrowing the throat further. Alcohol, especially late at night, relaxes the throat muscles, as do sleeping pills. If your partner has a distinct snoring pattern, regularly stopping snoring for about 20 to 30 seconds and waking up with a snort before starting to snore again, and if he or she also suffers from daytime tiredness, they need to seek medical advice. The first steps to deal with this are to lose weight and to cut down on alcohol, especially at night. Further treatment includes wearing a mask attached to a pump during the night which blows air into the throat. Sometimes surgery is recommended.

Pseudo-insomnia

Despite the name, this condition does not mean malingering. For example, people with pseudo-insomnia often fall asleep within twenty minutes of going to bed and get at least six hours' sleep. However, they feel as though they've hardly slept a wink all night. It seems that the quality of their sleep isn't deep enough for them to feel refreshed when they wake up in the morning. Most normal sleepers change positions 30 to 40 times during sleep and wake 4 or 5 times each night, but so briefly that they don't remember wakening. Lighter sleepers who are aware of these waking moments can feel that they've tossed and turned all night. When the brain waves of pseudo-insomniacs are monitored in sleep laboratories, some of them appear to be thinking all night while asleep. Some seem to spend the night dreaming that they are awake. One explanation that has been given for this is that their body functions remain active after they've fallen asleep, giving them the feeling of being awake.

Pain

Pain is a common cause of poor sleep. It often seems worse at night and chronic pain is very debilitating and depressing. If you know the cause of your physical pain and have been told that nothing can be done for its cause, you may consider getting your physician to refer you to a pain relief clinic or to a physiotherapist. Natural therapies can often relieve symptoms even though they may not be able to cure the cause of the pain.

In addition to the above medical conditions, sleep problems can also be attributed to the following.

Faulty body clocks

A few people have body clocks which are out of pace with the rest of the world. This can be detected through monitoring in sleep labs. Once people understand what the problem is they can sometimes adapt their lifestyle to fit in with their natural pattern. However, usually our lifestyle has to fit in with society's daytime working patterns. Sometimes people have a chronic inability to fall asleep until around 4–5am and then sleep well. However, if they have to get up the next morning, for example to go to work, they will always be short of sleep. They usually don't respond well to sleeping pills and don't appear to be suffering from any other sort of stress. There is apparently a difference in the mechanism regulating the day–night sleep cycle which triggers the time that they are ready for sleep.

Shift work and jet lag

This is often a cause of body-clock disturbance. Most people who have to go to bed in the morning and sleep until the afternoon take a week or ten days to adapt to the new pattern. The same applies to any change to the sleep–wake cycle, such as in jet lag. It is not just a person's sleep that has to adapt but the whole circadian rhythm involving the timing of hormone release and other bodily functions. Problems arise when working hours are regularly changed or when the shift worker tries to return to a normal pattern on a day or weekend off. If you have to work at night remember that your body clock needs at least a week to adjust to a new schedule.

In the following chapter we will be exploring the causes of insomnia. Once you understand the reasons for your insomnia there are many things you can do to improve your sleep. As soon as you decide on a plan of action to tackle your insomnia your sleep pattern will not only improve but you will also be well on the way to establishing a more satisfactory and fulfilling daytime life. As you read on, make a note of what applies to you and the steps you can take to regain control of your life.

CHAPTER 2

The Causes of Insomnia

There are many possible factors that can contribute to insomnia and we will be looking at some of these in detail in this chapter. First, however, the contributory factors associated with the three basic types of insomnia can be summarized as follows.

1 Taking a long time to get off to sleep

Factors that can contribute to this include:

- Habit.
- Stress. This may be at home or at work. Emotional stress includes anxiety, depression, unhappiness, anger, guilt.
- Unresolved problems.
- Certain medical conditions, neurological problems and psychiatric disturbances.
- Digestive problems and dietary factors. These include too much or too rich a diet late at night, stimulating food and drinks.
- Major life changes. These may be positive or negative changes and include bereavement, moving house, divorce, changing jobs, etc.
- Poor sleep routine. Napping during the day and needing less sleep than you think you do.

- Body-clock disturbances such as jet lag and shift work.
- External disturbances such as noise.

2   Waking during the night

The causes for intermittent sleep during the night include the above list plus frequent

- High anger and irritability.
- Heavy alcohol consumption. Withdrawal from alcohol or drugs – medically prescribed or otherwise.
- Nightmares. Fear of nightmares. Waking just before you are about to dream.
- Not being fully stretched during the day.

3   Waking early and not being able to go back to sleep

In addition to the factors in the first list are

- Severe depression.
- Sleeping-pill dependency.
- Alcoholism.

FOOD AND DRINK

Caffeine

A common cause of sleeplessness, caffeine is found in coffee, tea, chocolate and cola drinks. It is a drug on which many people develop a dependency. Although it is a well-known stimulant, some people drink ten or twenty cups of coffee or tea every day and are then surprised that they can't sleep well at night. As the body can process only so much at once, caffeine can remain in the system for several hours after drinking it. Not everyone is adversely affected by coffee but some studies show that when normal sleepers are given coffee late at night, it not only delays the onset of sleep by around 40 minutes but also affects the quality of sleep and performance of tasks the following day. If you have any difficulties sleeping you should cut down your intake of tea and coffee, especially during the evening.

Alcohol

People who regularly drink large amounts of alcohol tend to sleep lightly and wake early. Chronic alcoholics show similar sleep patterns to older persons, with frequent night-time awakenings, little or no delta sleep and decreased REM sleep. They also feel very sleepy during the day.

Allergies

Allergies to food and chemicals in food, drink, the atmosphere and furnishings can bring about many of the mood disturbances associated with insomnia, such as depression, anxiety and restlessness as well as physical symptoms.

Sudden weight loss and eating disorders

A sudden loss of weight through dieting, fasting or illness can temporarily disrupt sleeping patterns. Patients with eating disorders associated with the restriction of food intake, such as anorexia nervosa, tend to sleep little and wake often during the night. When anorexics start normal eating patterns and put on some weight, their sleep also returns to a more normal pattern.

LIFE CYCLE CHANGES

Babies and children

A newborn baby naturally causes a disruption in its parents' sleep pattern. Parents who accept that their sleep will be broken while the baby needs night-time feeds suffer less from tiredness than those who feel resentful. Feelings of resentment can also be picked up by the baby, thus making the problem worse. This is an especially tiring period for mothers. If possible take time when you can during the day to nap or simply to relax.

Children can also suffer from disturbed sleep and this in turn may disturb the sleep of their parents. A screaming baby or a bedtime struggle to get an older child to go to bed creates irritability which will affect your stress level during the day as well as at night. A regular, consistent routine that helps the child to understand it is bedtime should be established as early as possible. Severe problems would often not arise if they had been sorted out earlier on. You may wish to consider seeking more help in family therapy if your family problems seem too difficult or if you are confused by what is happening and need help in sorting it out. For practical advice dealing with specific problems of childhood the book *My Child Won't Sleep* by Jo Douglas and Naomi Richman is highly recommended.

Women and mid-life

The menopause can affect women's sleeping patterns as hormones adjust to biological changes and this often causes broken sleep. Night sweats can be an additional and uncomfortable cause of sleep disturbance. Sleep usually settles back into a pattern once the menopause is over, although due to the ageing process sleep may be lighter than it was before. For some women the menopause brings into focus other issues. These can include children leaving home – the 'empty-nest' syndrome – or having to face issues such as ageing and mortality. This can bring about further depression and anxiety. A positive approach during this phase is to view it as a new, challenging stage of life.

Ageing

As we get older the amount of sleep we need and the pattern of our sleep tends to change naturally. With increasing age we need less sleep. Many elderly people wake in the early hours of the morning, and because this didn't happen in their younger days they conclude they have – or are misdiagnosed as having – insomnia. As people grow older, many feel the need to nap during the day. Also, they have the time and opportunity to nap. This interferes with night-time sleep. On the simplest level, if your usual amount of sleep is seven hours a night, and you have gradually added a couple of hours of daytime napping, those two hours cut into your ration of seven hours' sleep. However, the effects of daytime napping are a bit more complicated than simply subtracting the amount of napping time from total night-time sleep. Napping during the day, especially during the early evening, often cuts more into our sleep ration than the actual time spent napping. No one quite knows the reason for this. However, it is a strategy that can be used creatively by people whose circumstances are such that they need extra waking hours.

It is also normal for older people to sleep more lightly than they once did, and to wake more often during the night. Everyone has brief moments of waking or near-waking during the night as they come out of REM cycles, but we don't usually remember them. As you get older those moments may turn into minutes. If you start worrying about it, that in itself will keep you awake. If you accept that this is a natural process and there is nothing wrong with you, you may begin to enjoy the experience of being awake but resting. Only start worrying if the minutes turn into hours, if you feel too miserable to enjoy them or if you are missing out on total sleep time (taking naps into account) and feel mentally and physically exhausted the next day. However, the fact that a changing sleep pattern is normal as we age doesn't mean that the elderly don't ever suffer from insomnia.

STRESS

Stress and daily life

Although 'stress' is a word we often hear these days there's a great deal of misunderstanding about what stress actually is. One reason for this is that there's a great difference between people in what they find to be stressful. Some experiences like mountain climbing or pot-holing can be fun for some people but frightening and stressful to others. Other experiences like the death of a loved one or divorce are stressful to all of us. Whether our life experiences lead to excitement, fear or an overwhelming sense of loss, we have to cope with them. In order to do this body and brain must have extra energy, and stress is the body's automatic and natural response which gives us this extra energy to meet our challenges. Events which can trigger stress may be short-lived, like a row with the boss, or long term, such as chronic illness, redundancy or bereavement. Stress can also be helpful as it often motivates us to do something when necessary.

In our daily lives there are situations and events which can make us anxious or stressful, and usually we can cope with most of these. However, the whole pattern of modern life makes greater and greater demands of us. To cope with these demands our human stress response goes into action, giving us extra power and energy when we need it. The danger is that we can overuse the stress response, with the result that our energy supplies will run down and both our health and ability to cope in our daily lives will suffer.

Anxiety and stress are part of the biological process called the 'arousal system'. When what arouses us is positive we call it pleasure or excitement, but when it's negative we call it unpleasant or stressful. For example, the thrill we feel when anticipating a pleasurable event, such as going to a party, we call excitement. If the event we are anticipating is a telling-off by our boss at work, we experience it as something unpleasant and call it stress even though the same biological processes are at work.

THE STRESS RESPONSE

Our stress response is vital, both to our survival as a species and to us as individuals trying to cope with our daily lives. Although some stress is essential to life, it can cause both mental and physical illness if we don't keep the correct balance. It is harmful when continuous states of crisis prevent the system from returning to normal (over-arousal) or when the system fails to react, as in a state of depression or apathy (under-arousal). Because it is crucial to survival the stress response can override many of our other human survival responses. If we keep the stress response on too high a pressure or keep it going for too long, the body will use its reserves to keep the stress response going at the expense of all the other body systems, including our defences to infections and illness. This can bring about serious biochemical changes.

Changes brought about by the stress response

When we're faced with a challenge in our daily lives the stress response instantly goes into action to give us the strength and energy we need. It's an intricate reflex involving that part of the brain called the hypothalamus, which triggers off a complex chain of chemical and nerve reactions and changes through the hormonal system and the sympathetic nervous system. The main changes are:

Heart and circulation

As the heart is stimulated there's an increase in heartbeat and pulse rate. There's an increase in the circulation of blood to the brain and to the limbs and a decrease of blood supply to the digestive system and skin where the blood vessels are constricted. Blood pressure is raised.

Lungs and breathing

Breathing becomes faster and more shallow using mainly the top of the lungs, which increases the possibility of hyperventilation.

Stomach, digestion and internal organs

Saliva dries up and our digestive system slows down. The blood that is usually involved in digestion is transferred to the limbs for quick action. Stores of fats and sugar are broken down and changed chemically to give us quicker strength and energy. Tension in the limb muscles is increased as they become geared up for instant action, but at the same time the muscles of the rectum and bladder relax.

All these changes bring about significant increases in energy, speed and strength. However, this is often far more than is necessary to meet the everyday challenges of living. If all these changes are not allowed to return to normal, strain will follow. At this point the symptoms of anxiety become more extreme and distressing and include those symptoms which lead doctors to prescribe tranquillizers. Severe symptoms can include panic attacks, breathlessness, rapid heartbeat, sweating, inability to concentrate, aches and pains and chronic insomnia.

SYMPTOMS OF STRESS

When people are stressed they can experience a whole range of unpleasant mental, emotional, physical and behavioural symptoms. Some people are more aware of these symptoms than others. What is important is that you recognize the way you personally respond to stress so that you can learn to control and prevent the symptoms.

Physical symptoms

When we have been tense for a long time – that is, suffering from chronic stress – this can bring about a general restlessness and can be seen in a whole variety of physical mannerisms, for example, knee-jiggling, nail-biting, etc. Physically, the muscles tense up. This is one of the first physical symptoms of stress and can result in a range of aches and pains felt in almost any part of the body – headaches, trembling hands, a stiff jaw and sensations such as a knot or butterflies in the stomach, or the throat muscles tensing up and making swallowing difficult. Tension in the bowel may result in either constipation or diarrhoea, or irritation to the bladder resulting in more frequent urination.

Other physical symptoms of stress include migraine, erratic breathing, hyperventilation, dizzy spells, sweating hands, cold fingers, dry mouth, numbness, increased heartrate, high blood pressure and chest palpitation. It can also lead to stomach ulcers, nausea and physical illness.

Emotional symptoms

Emotional symptoms of stress include feeling generally anxious, fearful or panicky, being moody or irritable or having angry outbursts. Other symptoms include feelings of depression, when we can feel tearful, hopeless, guilty, lonely, insecure, and can often be sensitive to criticism and feel misunderstood by others or resentful that others are against us.

Mental symptoms

Common examples of these are difficulty in concentrating and making decisions, forgetfulness, memory problems, tiredness, sensitivity to and feeling time pressure. Mental symptoms can be reflected in the way we think, such as depressed thinking (negative, self-critical thoughts), worrying (catastrophic thinking), difficulty in making rational judgements (distorted, irrational ideas) and making rash decisions when we are confused or muddled and get things out of perspective.

Behavioural symptoms

These symptoms involve the ways we try and bring down our excess energy and stress levels. These can sometimes lead to the abuse or over-use of substances like alcohol, drugs and cigarettes. People can develop mannerisms such as nail-biting and knee-jiggling or may generally neglect themselves or be accident-prone.

Behavioural changes can often be symptoms of stress – for example, when we eat or sleep less or more than usual or are more or less active than usual. Some people tend to work too much or too little, which can result in absenteeism when they have to take time off work. Some people become over-active socially and run about and talk too much, while others withdraw socially and avoid situations that make them anxious.

People are often bewildered and confused by their symptoms, sometimes worrying that they could be due to other, more serious physical causes. For example, symptoms of stress are pains in the head, stomach or in the chest area. If these symptoms continue, people can start thinking that their pain is because they have cancer or a brain tumour or that they are going to suffer a heart attack. As these symptoms can genuinely be due to causes other than stress, if you do suffer such aches and pains you should consult your family doctor. As in the following case of John, once you know that the cause of your pain is stress, try not to add to your stress levels by worrying unnecessarily.

When under stress, John suffered from chest pains which he immediately interpreted as the beginnings of a heart attack. This thought added to his anxiety and made the pain worse. Each time this happened he'd telephone for an ambulance and be admitted to the local hospital to be checked. Both his family doctor and the hospital staff became increasingly frustrated by what they saw as a hypochondriac wasting their valuable time and resources. Reassured by his family doctor after a thorough medical check-up, John attended a few sessions of stress management where he learned to recognize the symptoms of stress – which in his case included chest pain – and how to control them.

THE THREE STAGES OF STRESS

Stress is part of our general arousal system. At one end of the continuum, as we can see from the diagram overleaf, is the extreme of too little stress and at the other end strain and burn out. Before I go on to outline the three-stage model of stress, it can be seen from the diagram that under-arousal may also be distressing for us.

Stress Curve

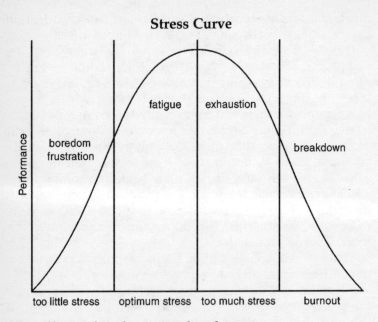

The effects of under-arousal and stress

To feel on top form physically and mentally we need to be at or around the optimum of the arousal curve. Too little stress makes us feel bored and frustrated. This feels uncomfortable so we often actively seek out situations – such as watching a movie or going to a football match – which stimulate or excite us to take us further up the arousal curve. These situations may be real events or we can use our imagination to create more stimulation.

We need challenges and satisfying goals in our daily lives in order to feel good. We usually find these in our work or hobbies. Ideally, work should be interesting and stimulating, and give us enough challenge to feel a sense of worth and achievement. However, not all of us are in the fortunate position where we are able to do interesting work. Worry and anxiety use more energy than being fully involved with a satisfying job and there is just as much illness from the stress of boredom and lack of fulfilment as there is from the anxiety of continual pressure. Frustration, aggression or apathy may result, leading to illness.

Stage 1: The beginning of stress

Any event or situation which is a physical or psychological challenge switches on our stress response to give us extra drive and physical and mental energy to cope with the situation. Only when the challenge is over will the stress response switch off. For example, if you're running to get the last train home a surge of energy enables you to race to the train with unexpected speed, and once you're on the train you relax and the stress response switches off. This first stage of stress doesn't last very long and isn't just essential to life but so familiar that we don't often recognize it as a stress response.

Stage 2: The maintenance of stress

Stage 2 stress is when stress is too much and/or goes on for too long. If stress is increased – for example, if the changes in our life are happening too suddenly or too quickly to allow us enough time to get used to them and adapt – we need to put more effort into coping. Similarly, if high levels of stress are kept going for too long, then our response to stress may begin to interfere with our ability to cope. For as long as a challenge lasts our stress response will continue to increase and produce energy, first by using up our available energy, then by using our energy stores and finally by breaking down fats and sugars stored in our organs and tissues. This results in the speeding up of all body functions to create the extra physical and mental energy that we need to meet the extra demands.

Just like the first stage of stress, this second stage is not necessarily bad unless we keep high levels of stress arousal going for too long. At this point any added problems, such as family or financial difficulties, job changes or pressures at work, overburden our coping system. When there's too much pressure on our arousal system we begin to experience warning signs, for example, irritability, impatience, sleeping difficulties, loss of concentration and depression. Often during this stage our work begins to suffer and we add to our stress by worrying about this, which pushes stress levels even higher and leads to the next stage of stress which is strain.

Stage 3: Strain

This is the end result when we have been under too much stress and/or it has gone on for too long and we have ignored the early warning signs. It is at this stage that damage is caused as too many demands are made on the mind and body without enough rest and sleep put back into the reserves. If we don't allow the body and brain to recuperate and the changes aren't reversed, when we try meeting any further demands we will experience strain. At this stage energy begins to flag and if we continue ignoring the symptoms of fatigue and stress we may reach a point where a breakdown in physical and mental health or 'burn-out' is likely. Typical complaints are loss of energy at work and at home. It is at this point that people say, 'I'm stressed.'

Recognition of strain

It is important to recognize symptoms of strain. The most common symptoms include the following.

Personality changes

When a person is under strain they often don't realize that they are strained. This is more often pointed out by friends and colleagues who recognize that the person is behaving differently from their usual self – for example, when a normally easygoing person becomes irritable and short-tempered or when a normally decisive person becomes confused and uncertain and gives contradictory orders as he or she tries to keep a grip on the situation.

Sleep patterns

Our sleep patterns become disrupted when we are under strain. It takes longer to get off to sleep and there is frequent wakening during the night and waking early in the morning. Worrying about not sleeping makes the situation worse, further preventing sleep and adding to the cycle of exhaustion. While some people are unable to sleep, others want to sleep more, and getting up in the morning may be difficult.

Seeking comfort

When we are under strain we often try and make things better by looking for comfort. However, this can often lead to the following destructive patterns.

Eating: While some people go off their food, others eat too much. Losing or putting on weight can be a sign of long-term stress.

Smoking and drinking: Many people smoke and drink to be sociable or because they enjoy it. It is also seen as a way of reducing anxiety and lifting depression. Although alcohol in moderation helps us relax and smoking temporarily lifts us, during stress we tend to rely on them more.

When we are exhausted, it becomes difficult to concentrate and we often become indecisive, irritable and short-tempered. If we ignore this or cover it up by drinking and smoking too much, we may gain temporary relief but we are just masking the problem and can end up feeling even worse. We may even lose perspective, feel depressed, oversensitive or withdraw from social activities.

In the long run, changes which result from strain must be taken seriously because corresponding biochemical changes in the body bring about high steroid levels which interfere with the immune system. At this stage people are vulnerable to any infection or illness and the weakest part of our system will break down first.

STRESS, STRAIN AND ILLNESS

Stress is often called a modern disease. In itself, it isn't a disease but a normal physiological response in order to help us fight illness and other crises or challenges with which we're faced. However, under certain conditions continued high levels of stress arousal can cause what we call stress-induced illness. Stress can also weaken the body and bring about the kind of conditions which allow illness or infection to develop. In this case we talk of stress-related illness, but the distinction between the two is often not as clear as this. In reality the relationship between stress and illness is very complex. The type of illness which develops from the strain of continuous high arousal depends partly on our genetic make-up and partly on the weakest link in our system at the time.

WHAT BRINGS ABOUT STRESS?

Stress may be brought about by something within ourselves – that is, an internal event such as some inner conflict or problem – or it may be triggered by something outside ourselves – an external event. But what causes one person stress may not cause another person stress. This is because we differ greatly in our needs – for example, in the time we need to finish a piece of work, the amount of food, relaxation and sleep that we need. This is because our personalities – that is, what we brought into the world with us, the care we had as children and the ways that we learned to cope with our experiences – are all different. For example, a person who's a perfectionist will have high standards for him- or herself, and will need more time to finish a task to his or her satisfaction than another person who may be able to rush through the same amount of work at twice the speed and not worry about it. If the same time limit is put on both of these types then the perfectionist or worrier will be the one who will be most vulnerable to stress.

Whether or not we experience a particular event as stressful will depend on an interaction of many factors. These include:

1   External events

These are the outside events that happen to us or the demands which are put on us. These can be short-lived – for example, meeting deadlines or giving an important presentation – or they can involve facing a threat, as when we narrowly avoid a car accident or someone questions our competence. External events can also be long term, such as the chronic illness of a loved one, bereavement or being made redundant at work. Even when our lives are going fairly smoothly we will, at some point or another, be faced with life's inevitable tragedies, triumphs and disasters. We may think that we're in control but really we have very little control over many of these external events that happen to us.

2   The amount and nature of change in our lives

The amount of change we experience in our lives and how we handle it affects how stressed we are and how we'll face stressful events. Stress itself is not a disease but it's a condition of our times and a part of life in a highly mobile technological society. Technological changes have been introduced to us both at home and in the workplace at a pace never witnessed before. All of them save time so that we're able to accomplish more and travel further in the space of a day than our grandparents could in weeks. However, we are the same species of people and haven't changed. So the question is – how do we cope and adapt to such a different pace of life?

A great deal of research has been carried out into the effect of change on our lives. A scale developed by Holmes and Rahe called 'The Social Readjustment Rating Scale' (1970) cites 43 stressful events in life. The scale gives each event a value according to the amount of adjustment we need to cope with that extra amount of change in addition to the events of our normal daily routine. Over the years the scale has been found to be a reliable and useful measurement of the effect of change on people in many different cultures. This scale is useful in assessing how much change an individual should allow in his or her life at any one time. Holmes and Rahe found that 80 per cent of people with over 300 points in one year ran the risk of illness in the near future. For those between 150 and 299 points, 50 per cent soon became ill, and of those with less than 150 point about 3 per cent became ill shortly after the life-event changes. This doesn't mean that illness will inevitably follow change – for example, one in five of those in the top bracket with very high scores for change don't become ill. Other factors have to be taken into account, such as the way which people cope with stressful situations. The experience of having had small problems to overcome and having coped successfully with them also has a positive effect on our ability to cope in the future.

Social Readjustment Rating Scale

rank	life event	value
1	Death of spouse	100
2	Divorce	73
3	Marital separation	65
4	Jail term	63
5	Death of a close family member	63
6	Personal injury or illness	53
7	Marriage	50
8	Fired at work	47
9	Marital reconciliation	45
10	Retirement	45
11	Change in health of family member	44
12	Pregnancy	40
13	Sexual difficulties	39
14	Gain of new family member	39
15	Business readjustment	39
16	Change in financial state	38
17	Death of a close friend	37
18	Change to different line of work	36
19	Change in number of arguments with spouse	35
20	Large mortgage	31
21	Foreclosure of mortgage or loan	30
22	Change in responsibilities at work	29
23	Son or daughter leaving home	29
24	Trouble with in-laws	29
25	Outstanding personal achievement	28
26	Wife begins or stops work	26
27	Begin or end school	26
28	Change in living conditions	25
29	Revision of personal habits	24
30	Trouble with boss	23
31	Change in work hours or conditions	20
32	Change in residence	20
33	Change in schools	20
34	Change in recreation	19

rank	life event	value
35	Change in church activities	19
36	Change in social activities	18
37	Small mortgage or loan	17
38	Change in sleeping habits	16
39	Change in number of family get-togethers	15
40	Change in eating habits	15
41	Vacation	13
42	Christmas	12
43	Minor violations of the law	11

3   Internal needs and beliefs

The way we respond to situations is different because we see them differently in the first place. It could even be said that we're not responding to the same situation. What one person views as an overwhelming threat may be perceived as a stimulating challenge to another person and a mere trifle to a third. It isn't the actual situation that causes us stress but the meaning that we attach to it that is different. Another reason we differ is that we experience stress – physically, mentally, emotionally and behaviourally – differently.

Stress can be brought about by our inner hopes, fears and beliefs as well as by our attitude to life – for example, the perfectionist who has to be perfect in all things. It can also result from struggling to meet the unrealistic expectations of other people as well as our own. For example, you may be expected to be a great manager when, in fact, you're a great practitioner but not very good at managing.

4   External support

Whether stress is triggered by external demands or by our own inner needs, the practical help or emotional support which others can give to us, whether at home or at work, can reduce the amount of stress we experience.

5   Control and predictability

We experience situations and events which we cannot control or predict as being more stressful than those which we can. The feeling of not being in control of one's future is very stress-inducing.

6   Our personal styles of coping

Whatever the situation is, whether or not it will be experienced as stressful will depend to some extent on our usual ways of coping with stressful situations. How we think we'll be able to cope with the situation also influences whether we'll experience stress. Because of our own personal experiences, training and expectation of ourselves and others, we react differently to events. For example, when faced with an identical situation, one person may conform, another may rebel and another try and change the situation. Yet another may not be affected by it at all.

People who are likely to suffer from under-arousal

- Housewives who are at home coping with small children under five are often under-aroused in spite of being very 'busy' all day. They are doing several jobs with different skills such as nanny, cook, gardener, nurse and housekeeper, whereas at the same time skills in which they may have been trained – work skills – cannot be practised. This itself can give rise to an underlying sense of frustration which is often not recognized as such. The lack of intellectual and social stimulation can also lead to feelings of isolation.

- The lonely, especially the elderly who if they have relatives may live too far away for frequent contact.
- People who work alone – for example, night-time caretakers and security officers, those working from home such as tele-workers, and single incapacitated people who live at home and who rely on other people for help.
- The retired whose lives may have focussed around work and who now find a large gap in their lives.
- People who have been made redundant and the unemployed. The latter have potential problems of identity as well as the loss of ability to practise their skills. In our modern industrial society people are often known for what work they do. When people lose their jobs they often experience a loss of self-respect and self-confidence.

People who are likely to suffer from over-arousal

- People who are ambitious and who drive themselves hard and fast to achieve top results in short time (the 'Type A' personality).
- People who double the amount of a normal day's work, such as a working wife and mother who has to juggle with the demands of a career and home responsibilities.
- People who start a business from scratch and give all their time and energy to the project seven days a week.
- People who have heavy responsibilities on top of a demanding job. These may be caring for a sick or handicapped child, or studying for further qualifications.
- People who give too much of themselves or who take on far too much.
- People who may not be overloaded but who over-react, treating every small incident as a major crisis.

STRESS, TIREDNESS AND SLEEP

We experience a state of normal tiredness when the body has used up its ready supply of energy and needs to rest in order to replenish and restore its balance. Usually at this point we naturally stop and rest. A difficulty is that often we have been taught from early childhood that we should make an effort, try hard and work to achieve goals. During this process we may have learned to take no notice of tiredness and so we don't pay attention to the body's signals. When we do eventually stop and sit down at the end of the day we are often surprised to find how tired we really are. It is helpful if we can recognize the different stages of tiredness and fatigue.

THE STAGES OF FATIGUE

1 Healthy tiredness

Healthy tiredness is a natural and normal reaction telling us when we need to stop or rest. This is when someone yawns, says they're tired and isn't worried about it, then decides on an early night or relaxing weekend. Work can be continued if need be although it takes more effort than usual. Your body and brain will be trying to tell you to cut out all non-essential work and you'll feel that you need to rest and reserve energy and resources.

2 Continuing tiredness

When tiredness continues beyond the first stage we reach the next stage when we're not able to shake off the feeling of tiredness. Often, at this second stage of tiredness, people complain about lack of energy, of being too tired at the end of the day to go out and do anything else, so that life becomes a round of work and sleep. When this happens a complete break from the usual routine is needed. This sort of tiredness may also be due to overload – for example, if you have a demanding job and evening chores and responsibilities, a demanding social life or difficulties at either home or work. Holidays give a chance for catching up with much-needed rest and sleep in order to restore the system to normal.

Sometimes this stage of tiredness is a sign that our mental and physical activities are out of balance. Those of us who work mentally and have little movement during the day need to redress the balance and build some form of physical exercise into our routine. It will help to remedy the chemical build-up which is causing the tiredness and reduce anxiety and lift depression. However, such new activity shouldn't be started if the tiredness is really that of exhaustion. We'll see how to note the difference later.

3   Exhaustion

At this point tiredness is at a dangerous level. People who have reached this level often don't even admit that they're tired. This is because they often become defensive and won't admit that there's anything wrong with them, although other people notice changes in their behaviour. Typically there are changes in their usual patterns, such as in their eating and sleeping habits.

Sleep patterns are altered in a variety of ways. When people are under strain they don't get enough sleep, usually because of difficulty in getting off to sleep together with waking early in the morning. At this stage people get frustrated quickly and flare up for very little reason. As a result personal relationships often deteriorate. Work suffers as the original, flexible thinking gives way to fixed ideas and set ways of doing things as the mind is closed to change. Leadership skills are affected and a person who was once a flexible, innovative leader becomes someone fixed in routine and bureaucracy.

Case study: Jim

Jim was the effective and well-liked boss of a small but extremely successful engineering company. Jim was happy with this state of affairs, although his partner was eager to expand the company. Due to the company's excellent track record, Jim's bank manager encouraged them to take out loans in order to expand. The company grew very rapidly, taking out further bank loans to finance taking on significantly more staff and expanding its premises.

Jim had coped well with the usual stresses of work when the company was a small, family-run concern. However, with growth came changes both in the organization and in the nature of work relations, which caused Jim additional stress. He began to experience symptoms of anxiety during the day, such as headaches, and slept poorly at night for the first time in his life. He tried to deal with his stress by drinking more alcohol at night. At first this helped, but eventually it led to even worse sleep as he woke often in the night and got up even more exhausted in the morning. It was with the final exhaustion stage that Jim's colleagues noticed a marked change in his personality. From being a typically easygoing, jovial man, flexible in what he demanded of his workforce, he became morose and quick to express his anger. The slightest deviation from the established pattern of working would throw him into a rage. In a relatively short time Jim had gone down the road from worry about work to increasingly severe stress levels and to his present state of strain.

CONTROLLING OUR STRESS LEVELS

The stress response has often been compared to the accelerator pedal of a car. If we find ourselves running late, we tend to push the accelerator to the floor. However, it's pointless putting our foot on the accelerator while we're sitting in a traffic jam. If we allow ourselves to become stressed by circumstances that are similarly beyond our control, the extra energy will only be diverted into tension, anxiety and frustration. Sometimes we just need to accept things for what they are.

Coping with stress involves driving oneself sensibly by understanding and paying attention to the stress response and its symptoms. In this way can prevent a great deal of strain and illness. In later chapters we'll be looking at ways in which we can cope better with anxiety and stress. But first we'll look at some practical steps we can take to tackle insomnia.

CHAPTER 3

How to Overcome Insomnia

RESTORING A BETTER SLEEP PATTERN

Exercise

Some light exercise in the early evening can release energy and tension. Exercise can also help restore the balance if you've spent most of the day being physically inactive. However, avoid taking exercise late at night, which over-stimulates the body. The simple answer is to exercise earlier in the day – the best times for strenuous exercise are the afternoon and early evening. To help with insomnia a light walk to unwind last thing at night is helpful.

Naps

While you are recovering a normal sleep pattern, naps are best avoided. The exceptions include the parents of new babies, who are not technically insomniacs but are likely to be getting broken sleep. If you're elderly and the need for a daytime nap feels overpowering, remember that if you take a nap you need to allow for less sleep at night.

You can overcome daytime sleepiness, especially after lunch, with some deep breathing or a brisk walk. Try not to fall asleep in the chair watching television in the evening. You'll only have to wake up again in order to go to bed, which is confusing for your body clock and makes it more difficult to get off to sleep again.

Sleeping pills

An occasional sleeping pill taken on your doctor's advice may be useful to help you to get over a specific crisis and re-establish your sleep pattern. However, these days most doctors are very aware of the dangers of the long-term use of sleeping pills. The main reasons for this are:

1   Their effects wear off after a few weeks, which can lead people to take higher and higher doses as their effectiveness lessens.
2   Long-term use can lead to physical and/or psychological dependence.
3   They can have unpleasant side-effects – for example, some people feel anxious or even low in spirits when taking the pills.
4   They can lead you to lose confidence in your own ability to cope.
5   They can dampen positive feelings (such as pleasure) as well as negative feelings.
6   When people try to stop taking the pills they sometimes suffer unpleasant symptoms (withdrawal effects), including anxiety.
7   Sleeping pills don't solve the original problem which caused you not to sleep in the first place.

Sleeping pills can take you into a vicious cycle of physical and/or psychological dependence when taken over a prolonged period. This is because your body builds up a tolerance to the drug after a few weeks, which means that the dose you were initially taking becomes ineffective and you sleep less. The temptation then is to take more pills to help you to sleep, and so on. In the long run they can hinder sleep rather than solve the problem of why you can't sleep.

Coming off sleeping pills

Many people who've been taking sleeping pills for months or even years are now being encouraged to come off them, and alternative ways of dealing with life's problems are being used. To try living without sleeping tablets is to give you a new challenge. Never stop taking them suddenly – a steady and gradual reduction is best at a pace with which you feel comfortable. Some people withdraw easily while others have more difficulty. It is important that before you start withdrawing you find out what is right for you.

1 Tell your doctor that you wish to come off sleeping pills. If possible try and work out a personal withdrawal plan with your doctor. The doctor might refer you on to a professional who is experienced in helping people withdraw from medication – such as a clinical psychologist – and together you can explore better ways of coping.
2 Some people find it useful to tell their family and friends of their decision and to ask for their support and understanding when withdrawing.
3 Many people find it helpful to find the support of other people who've been through the difficulties of withdrawing from sleeping pills and tranquillizers. Try finding out about self-help groups in your area. Self-help groups can help in the sharing of problems, discovering that you are not alone and can help provide you with information and help you start looking at why you started taking the tablets in the first place, as well as giving advice, encouragement and support in withdrawing from the pills.

When you have decided to stop:

- Congratulate yourself.
- Withdraw from tablets gradually.
- Reward yourself for each step, however small.

Withdrawal effects

When you try to stop taking sleeping pills you may be tempted to cut down too quickly or by too big a dose, or even to suddenly stop them completely. If you do this you can suffer from very uncomfortable withdrawal effects, which may even lead you to think that you have an underlying problem or illness that is somehow controlled by the pills. This is why it is important to withdraw very gradually, tapering off the dosage over at least three months if not longer. The worst withdrawals happen when people give them up suddenly.

Withdrawal effects can include anxiety-related symptoms such as feeling panicky, tense, restless and difficulty in sleeping. It is important to realize that these withdrawal effects, which include 'rebound insomnia' – the insomnia caused by your body craving the drug – are the result of the sleeping tablets themselves and are not necessarily a recurrence of the original cause of sleeplessness or a sign of an underlying sleep problem.

Sometimes the original anxieties for which the tablets were initially prescribed resurface. This is easier to cope with if you see this as part of the healing process rather than a sign of illness. Counselling from a professional or alternative practitioner can help you through this stage. Practitioners of natural therapies can be very supportive in helping you to come off sleeping pills and dealing with the after-effects including detoxifying the body. If you're seeking additional treatment for your insomnia it's a good idea to let your family doctor know.

Herbal sedatives

Alternative therapists would much rather help you solve sleeping problems than be dependent on medication, but herbal tranquillizers can be useful and safe as a temporary aid to help you recover your normal sleep.

There's a wide range of sedative herbal pills which can be bought over the counter at health-food shops and some chemists. Most of them contain slightly differing proportions of the same ingredients, including valerian, scullcap, passiflora, wild lettuce and other sleep-inducing herbs. They can often be taken during the day to counteract anxiety as well as to help you sleep at night.

Herbal pills don't have the same side-effects as conventional sleeping pills. Occasionally a person may have an individual allergic reaction to a herbal product, but this doesn't compare with the thousands of people suffering from tranquillizer addiction and withdrawal symptoms. Most herbal remedies are mild and aren't technically addictive physically. However, it is possible to become psychologically dependent on them or use them as a substitute for dealing with the causes of your insomnia. Taken regularly for a few weeks their effect is reduced.

Food and drink

The timing of meals

When we eat is as important as what we eat. Natural practitioners recommend a large breakfast, a moderate lunch and a light supper, eaten preferably no later than 6pm. There are biological reasons for this. The human digestive system functions best in the morning, and gets slower throughout the day. This means that food eaten late in the evening is liable to remain in the stomach half-digested during the night and can thus interfere with good sleep.

Sometimes it can contribute to a build-up of toxins which leads to poor health.

Now may be a time when you wish to change your eating habits to encourage your body to relax and sleep. However, it's important to remember that establishing a new routine doesn't mean that you have to keep rigidly to the rules. For example, if you're invited out to dinner later than your usual mealtime, you can adapt by keeping the portions and alcohol down. The important thing is to relax and enjoy it. Relaxing when you eat is probably just as important as when you eat.

Food

Foods to avoid in the evening include those which fill you up and overwork the digestive system without giving your body any real fuel – for example, refined carbohydrates such as white flour and sugar. Remember sugar is contained in a whole range of foods including, of course, cakes, chocolates and biscuits.

Processed foods are also best avoided. We have become increasingly aware of the effects of chemical additives in food, but many processed foods contain additives to which some people have an adverse reaction without always realizing the cause of it. High-fat foods also put a strain on the digestive system when eaten in the evening – so there may well be truth in the myth that cheese causes nightmares.

Stimulating foods that can keep us awake also include raw vegetables, salads and fruits so naturopaths recommend fruit and/or dried fruit with breakfast and a large raw salad with lunch. Be careful of the amount of salt you use in cooking as well as the amount you add once the food is on your plate – too much salt raises the blood pressure and puts the body into overdrive.

Root vegetables are believed by naturopaths to be more sedative than those growing above the ground. Also sedative are the unrefined carbohydrates – potatoes, wholegrain bread, pasta and rice – so these are best eaten with the evening meal. Many foods, when combined with carbo-hydrates, lead to the production of an amino acid called tryptophan, which is the main building block for serotonin. Serotonin is a neuro-chemical which helps sleep. Foods in this category include milk, eggs, meat, nuts, fish, hard cheeses, bananas and pulses.

Some people recommend eating a light snack containing tryptophan last thing at night, such as a bowl of cereal or a banana, to ward off night hunger. However, this is a deci-sion you must make for yourself. Night is the time when the body should be ready for sleep, not digesting food. If a late-night snack suits you and helps you sleep, that may be the most important factor while you recover a sleep pattern.

Drink

A warm bedtime drink can be soothing and comforting, but make sure you don't drink too much late in the evening. Many elderly people complain of having to get up to go to the bathroom during the night without connecting it with their late-night drinks. As we get older our kidneys become more active during the night so the amount we can drink before bedtime will be less than we could drink when we were younger. If this is a problem, try having your drink no later than an hour before bedtime.

The tradition of having a hot milky drink at bedtime is probably based on the fact that milk contains both trypto-phan and calcium, which is a muscle relaxant and soothing to the nervous system. A cup of hot milk accompanied by calcium and magnesium supplements can help you get off to sleep, especially if you suffer from restless legs syndrome. However, not all milky drinks are good for sleep – chocolate has a high caffeine content. Plain hot milk or malted milk are best. A sprinkling of nutmeg on top is also said to be sleep-inducing. Some people find milk hard to digest, and as it is a food in its own right dietary purists would not recommend it last thing at night. Others find cider vinegar and honey helps them to sleep. The mixture contains a good supply of trace elements including calcium. A teaspoonful of each should be taken in a small cup of boiling water. If your sleeplessness is related to indigestion, slippery elm makes a soothing drink.

Avoid coffee and tea in the evening as these are stimulants and can keep you awake. If you suffer from insomnia try drinking herbal teas, spring water and pure fruit juices instead. If you have difficulty giving up coffee altogether try substituting with non-caffeine drinks that you can buy in health-food stores such as dandelion coffee or cereal drinks. (Herbal drinks are dealt with in more detail in Chapter 7, under 'Medical Herbalism'.)

Alcohol

A little alcohol acts as a relaxant and can help you sleep, but drinking every night and heavy drinking disturb sleep and cause early waking or lead to dependency and thus bring about even more problems. Passing out through drink is not sleep! You should also be aware that although alcohol may help you to get off to sleep initially, it can cause insomnia. To digest alcohol your liver and kidneys have to work extra hard, and your body has to provide extra adrenalin which is a stimulant. It has also been found that alcohol reduces REM sleep.

Allergies and sensitivities

Most people know about it if they are suffering from a food allergy. However, intolerances are usually more difficult to pinpoint. Some people are sensitive to particular foods without having a complete allergic reaction. The degree of sensitivity can also vary, with a reaction only happening or intensifying when people are stressed. The substances which most commonly cause allergic reaction or intolerance are wheat, eggs, dairy products, sugar, coffee, chocolate and oranges, as well as certain chemicals and additives.

Start noticing your reactions to foods and drinks, especially those that you crave or consume every day. If you notice that you regularly feel extra hyped-up or low after any particular food or drink, try cutting it out of your diet for a week or so and see whether this makes any difference. If you are allergic or intolerant you may get withdrawal symptoms, such as headaches or nausea. If this happens to you, tell yourself it is really a good sign because it shows that your system is reacting and cleansing itself of something that was doing it harm.

Supplements

Experts' views on the value of vitamin and mineral supplements vary greatly, especially between orthodox medical doctors and natural therapists. The general medical opinion is that as long as you eat a healthy, balanced diet you don't need to add anything else. However, natural therapists point out that so much of our food is affected by things such as pesticides, pollution and preservatives that most people's vitamin and mineral intakes need adding to. This is particularly so when someone is stressed, as is often the case with insomniacs.

Supplements are only useful when they supply what you are short of. Taking more of a vitamin or mineral than you actually need is wasteful and can in some cases be harmful. Because of the increasingly confusing range of vitamins, minerals, herbal remedies and more exotic supplements in health-food shops, advice from a nutritionist, homeopath or naturopath can help clarify your individual needs and save you unnecessary expense on useless or unproved supplements.

Noise

Loud noises disturb sleep. This is natural, and is built into us as a species because loud or unexpected noises often signify danger and we need to be awake and alert to deal with it. Our sensitivity to noise varies. Some people can sleep through a party but wake when their baby cries. People who sleep near excessive noise should try to lessen the sound. Loud noise, such as aircraft or busy streets, can interfere with restful sleep, even in people who don't wake up and who can't remember the noise the following morning. People who sleep near excessive noise should try heavy curtains in their bedrooms or use earplugs to protect the amount of restful sleep they do get. Earplugs are particularly useful in muffling disturbing sounds if the noise is very near you, such as the sound of your partner snoring in bed. Heavy curtains can also block out bothersome light.

Often it isn't the noise itself but the quality of it – how we interpret and experience it – that makes it unpleasant. For example, when measured in decibels the sound of waves crashing on a shore or the sound of a waterfall would be as loud as troublesome traffic noise, but many people find these sounds soothing and sleep-inducing. Some people find that they can cope better with annoying outside noise by creating their own kind of background noise – listening to soothing music through headphones or having the radio on softly at the bedside can help to block out intrusive noise.

Anticipating noise

Freud pointed out that when we are anxious, unhappy or afraid we are more sensitive to noise. In this way a cycle can be set up. Anticipating noise can make you anxious and prevent you from sleeping. When the noise does happen you'll be even more sensitive to it, experiencing it as being louder than you would normally.

Noisy neighbours

Noisy neighbours can be infuriating, and getting angry is going to keep you awake just as much as the noise. Very often the problem is as much to do with bad soundproofing as the actual level of noise, particularly in apartments. If you can't do anything about improving your soundproofing and the noise is regular and loud, tell the neighbours about it calmly. If you don't already know them, forming friendly relations with the person causing the noise can make the disturbance less threatening and some negotiation possible. Your attitude can make a lot of difference to how badly you're disturbed. Telling yourself that you're being disturbed by nasty inconsiderate people will make it worse.

The next time noise starts up just as you are going to sleep, you have a choice. You can get angry and tense, or you can try and cope with it differently. Try, for example, bearing with the noise without attaching to it any emotional thoughts about other people's selfishness. Relax your body, breathe deeply and regularly. Know that you're getting the physical rest you need and thus reduce your anxiety. Getting worked up about it only makes insomnia more likely.

A soothing bedroom

Your bedroom should be warm and welcoming with a peaceful atmosphere.

Colours

Colours not only influence our visual senses, they also affect us individually – we find some colours are stimulating, others calming.

The bed

Your bed should be comfortable, ideally with a firm but not over-hard mattress. Soft mattresses aren't good for your back. It is best to sleep with a single pillow which keeps your neck at a more natural angle. Some people find hop- or herb-filled pillows help them to sleep. You can get these at many health shops.

Fresh air

The room you sleep in should be set at a moderate temperature – not too hot and not too cold. You'll wake up at night if you are either too warm or too cold. There should be some circulation of fresh air provided it doesn't make the room too cold. If you don't like sleeping with an open window try leaving it open for a while before going to bed.

Natural fabrics

Over the last few years complaints such as headaches, depression, stress, rashes and nausea have been related to factors like artificial lighting, air-conditioning, windows that you can't open and static electricity from synthetic furniture and fabrics. Some of these factors can affect your home, particularly if you are sensitive to them. An increasing number of synthetic fabrics are used in furnishings, bed linen and nightclothes so try natural fabrics in your bedroom.

TACKLING THE HABIT OF INSOMNIA

Keeping a sleep diary

One of the first steps in tackling insomnia is to find out how much sleep you actually do get at night – estimates we make the following morning of our night's sleep are notoriously inaccurate. One way of finding out both how much sleep you get and your sleep pattern is to keep a sleep diary for at least two weeks. This may be a bothersome task to begin with, but do keep it up. It will be worth it if it helps you overcome insomnia. By keeping the diary you can also find out if any daytime events affected your sleep at night.

To make your sleep diary mark a sheet of paper as in the diagram overleaf – and keep the diary and a pencil next to your bed. You may be able to use an existing light such as the light of the alarm clock, or you may wish to use a small nightlight or torch. First record what time you go to bed. After you've gone to bed place a tick in the box every ten minutes throughout the night. If you miss a ten-minute stage then you've been asleep. Knowing this may help you to worry less and sleep better. Record what time you wake up in the morning and then the time you get up. Now you have a complete record of your night's sleep. From the diary you can then add up the times that you were awake during the night and subtract it from your total sleep time.

The 'stimulus control' method

A successful way of treating habitual or 'conditioned' insomnia is a technique used in behavioural psychology called 'stimulus control'. The procedure, which consists of a series of guidelines outlined below, teaches you how to associate bed and bedtime with sleep and sleep alone.

1 Use your bed and bedroom for sleep and sex only.
2 Always get up at the same time, including weekends and holidays. You may be tempted to lie in but if you take more sleep than you need it will be more difficult to get off to sleep the following night.
3 Don't take naps during the day.
4 Don't go to bed until you're really sleepy.

Sleep Diary

WEEK 1

Medication	Date (night of)	Time to bed	Time awake in night	Time awake in morning	Totals	Comments

5 If you haven't fallen asleep within twenty minutes of being in bed, don't stay there tossing and turning but get up and do something else in another room. Don't go back to bed until you're ready to fall asleep. The same applies if you wake up in the middle of the night for more than ten minutes or so. Don't associate your bedroom with lying awake.

6 Don't let your worries about not sleeping add further to your anxiety and prevent you from sleeping.

GETTING READY FOR SLEEP

Making a clear division between daytime and night-time activities

Try and make a clear division between your daytime and night-time activities well before you go to bed. Daytime hours are for action and activity, while night-time hours are for rest and relaxation. Sleep doesn't come when the mind is alert and occupied with the problems of the day, nor to a body tensed up and ready for action. Establish a separate winding-down period in the evening. If you just can't manage a clear stop to day- and work-related activities at the end of the normal working day, then at least try and set aside two hours for a separate 'evening time' before you go to bed.

At night your mind should be focussed away from the problems of the day. It needs to be occupied, but in soothing, pleasurable and gentle activities after a working day, so try and avoid too much mental stimulation during the evening, such as talking about family problems or job plans, or working late into the night. Find out what helps you personally switch off from daytime concerns and relax. Do things that you enjoy, such as talking to friends, being with your family, reading or other hobbies that help you relax. Some people find it helpful to wind down by watching television, but passively watching television doesn't work as well as listening to music, reading or relaxing with friends. Diversion is important as just passively relaxing may only mask problems and worries which can flood back as soon as the passive activity stops.

If you find it difficult to switch off daytime worries, try writing a list of all the problems that are on your mind and then plan to tackle them the next day, not worry about them during the evening. Write them all down on a piece of paper so that if more come to your mind during the course of the evening you can add them to the list. If you need to have difficult family discussions, get them over with early on in the evening. If matters aren't resolved write down what is left that needs sorting out and make a definite time to continue the discussion another time and not in bed. The same applies to anything else that may be worrying you. Write it down, along with any decisions you may have made about dealing with it, then put it away for the day.

ESTABLISHING A GOOD BEDTIME ROUTINE

It is important, especially if you have been suffering from insomnia for some time, to create a regular bedtime routine. As we've seen from the stimulus-control programme, this means establishing a distinct time for bed and sleep. Keep your bedtime as regular as possible, even if that means giving up the end of an interesting television programme. Try and go to bed at the same time every night and get up at the same time, even though you may have slept poorly the night before. Be strict about this, especially at weekends when you may be tempted to sleep in. This may be difficult at first when your new routine may involve you going to bed when you don't feel sleepy and you wake up feeling tired and longing for 'just a few minutes more' in bed. However, tackling the problem of insomnia is like any other learning or training in a new skill. You may need a few weeks or so for both body and mind to get used to the new pattern and what seemed so difficult at first becomes easier. If you find waking up very difficult, one strategy is to put a very loud alarm clock on the other side of the room before you go to bed so that you have to get up to turn it off. When you wake put the light on immediately and turn on a radio.

The stimulus-control programme emphasizes that the bedroom is only for sleep. Don't watch television, listen to the radio, write letters, work, smoke or eat or drink in bed. The one exception is sex – you can engage in sexual activities in bed without disrupting normal sleep patterns. By reserving the bed for sleep and sex only you'll no longer associate it with wakeful activities. The mere act of getting into bed will send a message to your mind and body that it's time to go to sleep. However, some people find reading in bed takes their minds away from the worries of the day and helps them sleep. When you're trying to train yourself for better sleep it's important to stick to the system you chose for a proper trial. If you've chosen the stimulus-control programme, stay with it for at least a month before trying something else.

Winding down the mind

Having made a clear division between day- and night-time activities, create a regular bedtime routine of winding down mentally and physically during the hour or so before you go to bed. Make it a time for letting go of the day and its stresses. Do things which you enjoy, such as reading quietly or listening to some of your favourite music.

Relaxing the body

It's important that both your body and mind are relaxed before going to bed so a clear division should be made between day and night-time for the body, too. Avoid strenuous physical exercise during the evening. It can over-arouse you and prevent sleep. However, if you've been generally physically inactive during the day, some light exercise can be helpful as it releases physical and mental tension. For example, a restful walk can help you relax if you've been cooped up all day.

You may find doing some relaxation exercises during the evening helps your body to get rid of tensions and get ready for sleep. Try the following exercise to practise moving from one state to the other.

Relaxation exercise

Breathe gently and slowly, breathing out more fully than you are aware of breathing in. Let the chest fill with air naturally without effort on your part, but be aware of breathing out fully. On each out-breath feel your 'readiness for action' flowing out. Start with the thighs and legs and feel them gradually getting heavier and warmer with every out-breath. Slowly achieve the effect in every muscle of the body, feeling and enjoying the warmth and heaviness which is left as all tension drains away.

Feel your back, shoulders, head and pelvis sinking further and further into the bed as you continue breathing gently and slowly. Gradually quieten the breathing until it's inaudible and you are still. Try not to think about sleep at all. In the above warm, heavy and relaxed still state, sleep will follow naturally.

Bath

A warm bath in the evening is relaxing and can relieve the physical and mental stresses of the day and help you sleep.

Make the bath warm, but not too hot. Take your bath at least an hour or so before bedtime as a hot bath, especially taken late at night, may have the opposite effect and wake you up. A bath is especially pleasant and sleep-inducing with herbal or aromatherapy preparations. Suitable aromatherapy oils include lavender, camomile and hops. Allow yourself time to soak so that you get the full, soothing benefit while you relax, breathing in the vapour while your body absorbs the oils.

TAKING CHARGE OF WORRYING AND ENCOURAGING BETTER SLEEP

Worrying can be useful during the day because it's a process we use to solve problems. However, you can't wind down and get into a restful state ready for sleep if you go to bed worrying about the problems of the day gone by or trying to sort out the problems of the next day. Night-time is not the time to deal with anxieties, regrets and sorting out difficulties. For good sleep at night it's important to deal with unfinished business during the day. Once you start taking some sort of action, even if it's only deciding to act, it will be a start to tackling the problem during the day rather than letting your mind worry about it at night.

Some people aren't particularly worried about anything but just have very active minds. Many accept this and often quite comfortably use the time they lie awake in coming up with ideas and plans. However, others find their thoughts are unpleasant, sad or anxious. Instead of being in a state ready for sleep, your mind replays past regrets, missed opportunities or lost happiness. These need to be dealt with, but bed is not the right place for this. Talking to someone – whether a friend, partner, or professional counsellor – about your problems is a good start to helping you deal with them.

TECHNIQUES FOR DEALING WITH NIGHT-TIME WORRYING

Self-talk

One of the best ways to break unhelpful habits is to start replacing them with helpful ones. The first thing is to recognize in what particular ways your habitual thinking or behaviour is maintaining your poor sleep. How do you talk to yourself and others about your sleep? If you label yourself 'insomniac' and tell yourself every time you go to bed that you'll never be able to go off to sleep, you are simply reinforcing the habit that keeps you awake. You can change some of that thinking by telling yourself that you are now on the way to improving your sleep and no longer keep saying to yourself and others that you are an insomniac.

Although it may be difficult to acknowledge, there is sometimes something to be gained by having insomnia. Psychologists call this a 'secondary gain' – for example, when a child is 'ill' in order to gain their parents' love and attention. Similarly, insomnia may prevent people from having to face up to other problems, take up new challenges or anything else which might mean change. This does not mean they are choosing to sleep badly on purpose, but there might be a secondary gain for them. If you think this could apply to you, try the following exercise.

Self-talk exercise

First, close your eyes and imagine saying to yourself and your family and work colleagues how well you sleep. How do you feel when you say this? Now imagine how different your life would be, how different you would be and what other people's reactions to you would be like. To begin with such statements will probably feel uncomfortable because they are not true.

Start noticing your habitual thoughts about insomnia. In particular, look out for sentences beginning, 'I always' or 'I never' – for example, 'I always wake up tired', 'I always wake up for hours in the middle of the night' or 'I'm never going to get to sleep tonight'. Although they may feel true to you they may not actually be true.

Monitor all your sleep-related thoughts and write them down. Many of the thoughts will be so automatic that it often takes time to notice you are thinking them at all. Once you know what they are you can challenge them and replace them with more helpful thoughts. This is the next step – replacing your negative statements with positive ones.

Positive sleep statements might be 'I'm now learning how to sleep better' or 'better sleep will come in time'. Make sure your new statements are ones that you can believe. Going to the other extreme by telling yourself 'I'm going to sleep perfectly tonight' may not work. It may simply create more tension, whereas a statement such as 'I will just take tonight for a start' may well lead you to sleep better that night.

The process of changing is: notice – stop – change

Notice what you say to yourself and start looking at your beliefs about both your sleep and yourself.
Stop thinking of yourself as insomniac and start seeing yourself as well on the way to good sleep.
Change your self-talk. Once you realize that you have some control over your thinking and your reactions to these thought patterns, many of the obstacles to good sleep will get less.

Distraction

Distraction is one of the most helpful techniques for diverting the mind from worrying. If your body is relaxed but your mind is still active and prevents you from sleeping, train yourself to focus on something else.

One method of distraction is to make up mental tasks which will keep your mind occupied and bored enough so you drop off to sleep. These include the old remedies like counting sheep, counting backwards from 200 or listing in alphabetical order the names of books or flowers. Alternatively, you can mentally recite to yourself a verse of a poem or the lines of a song over and over again.

Listening to the radio has been the salvation of many insomniacs. For some people, however, this has a disadvantage in that if there is a really interesting programme they may be over-stimulated and stay awake to hear it.

If worrying thoughts come into your head, try just letting them go, knowing that you will deal with them at a more appropriate time. If they persist write them down and then leave them. Concentrate on your breathing. As you breathe in think of calm, peace and tranquillity – and then breathe out and just let the worry go.

Using mental images

A useful technique that can help you sleep is to use images to activate the alpha waves that precede sleep. For example, you could imagine or remember a particularly pleasurable scene or go through a film that you enjoyed.

Listening to your thoughts

Another way of dealing with negative or anxious thoughts is not to resist them but to listen to them in an objective way, as though you are listening to a radio programme, rather than drumming up energy in trying to find solutions to them. Remember, the less anxious and the more pleasant your thoughts, the more likely you are to relax and get off to sleep.

TECHNIQUES FOR DEALING WITH SPECIFIC NIGHT-TIME WORRIES

If you're being kept awake by specific problems, learn to deal with them during the day so that you don't take unfinished business to bed with you. Find some time during the day or early evening to write a list of the worries or anxieties that are keeping you awake. Once you've spotted the problem, write down what you can do about it. If you're worried about a job interview, work out the steps you can take to prepare yourself for it. If getting a job interview is difficult – what can you do about it? Think about alternative courses of action that you can take. Let your mind wander and see what alternatives it can come up with.

A technique that is useful is rehearsal through the use of the imagination. Try out the following technique. Once you've decided on your course of action, close your eyes for a few minutes and see yourself taking it. If you're anxious about some event coming up, picture yourself dealing with it calmly and well. Try not to picture all the difficulties that can be put in your way. Set the scene very clearly. See yourself with your problem solved, or having achieved the thing you've dreaded doing. Imagine telling someone about it and hearing their praise. Don't worry if you can't visualize it clearly but try and get some sort of picture. Imagine how you'll feel – relieved, pleased with yourself, no longer anxious. In this way you're teaching your mind that solutions are possible and that anxiety or hesitation or procrastination aren't the only options open to you. Then close your notebook and put it in a drawer for the night – or leave it downstairs – so that you go to bed knowing that you've done everything you can. Physically putting your list away tells your anxiety that that's it for today.

Thought-stopping and breath-counting to silence worries

If you find yourself going over and over the same worries instead of dropping off to sleep, mentally shout 'Stop!' to yourself, give yourself a pinch and focus intensely on your breathing. Breathe slowly and smoothly, counting each time you breathe in and each time you breathe out – 'breathe in one, breathe out two, breathe in three, breathe out four', and so on. Each time the worries intrude on your counting, repeat the 'Stop!' and start counting breaths over again. Focus on the here-and-now and your breathing.

GOING TO BED AND NOT BEING ABLE TO SLEEP

By using the stimulus-control programme you can train yourself to accept that bed is the place for body and mind to relax and let go. Get your body in as comfortable a position as possible and know that your mind will soon be taking you into sleep. Don't *try* to get to sleep. Rather know that you've done all the right things to bring about good sleep and sleep will come in its own good time. Even a good sleeper takes on average 15 minutes or so to get off to sleep. If you're still awake after 20 minutes, get up, go into a different room and do something – have a small warm drink, read, write a letter – until you feel drowsy enough to return to bed. The same applies if you wake up in the middle of the night. The worst thing you can do is to lie in bed tossing and turning, worrying or brooding. One patient kept her ironing to do for such occasions. This was a task she disliked and she found that as soon as she set up the ironing board to start ironing at night drowsiness soon overcame her! Some people who find that they are at their most creative at night welcome the opportunity for this extra time and don't miss their sleep.

LEARNING TO COPE WITH NIGHT-TIME WAKING

Try not to worry if you occasionally wake up during the night. If you do wake up and start worrying about it you'll become even more alert and find it more difficult to get back to sleep. This then confirms your belief that you can't sleep. After a while you may become sensitized to normal night-time waking, becoming quickly alert and finding it difficult to go back to sleep despite trying. This is how the problem of night-time waking begins. The problem is then maintained or made worse as you begin to anticipate waking up in the night, worry about it and become increasingly concerned about being tired the next morning. It is important to remember that you are still resting if you are aware of being awake but feel drowsy and relaxed.

If you do wake up during the night and find it difficult to go back to sleep, rather than lying in bed tossing and turning it is best to get out of bed. Preferably, move to another room and do something distracting and restful until you begin to feel sleepy and return to bed. Some people find it helpful to do crossword puzzles or knit while others prefer to listen to the radio or to some soothing music. It is important for you to find the distracting activity that is right for you. It should be something that isn't too demanding because that over-stimulates you and keeps you too alert for sleep. If you find your mind keeps churning over problems or thinking about things you have to do the next day, a good idea is to adapt the 'worry list' or 'to-do list' that was used for dealing with problems during the winding-down period prior to going to bed. Some find it helpful to keep the list by the bedside so that when a worry comes to mind they add it to the list to be dealt with in the morning.

The two-hourly sleep rhythms: go with the flow!

The periods of deep sleep and light sleep alternate about every two hours, although this can vary between individuals. If you wake during the night and stay awake, don't stay awake worrying. Get up and make a hot drink. You have plenty of time before the next two-hour period of deep sleep is due. When you feel drowsy go back to bed and settle down again, getting warm and heavy as before and concentrate not on sleep but on becoming as quietly relaxed as possible in order that the body's work of rest and repair is still going on. In this state sleep naturally follows the body's natural two-hour rhythm of deep sleep periods.

OTHER STRATEGIES FOR OVERCOMING INSOMNIA

Paradoxical intention

If you've tried all the usual ways of coping with insomnia outlined in this chapter and have met with little success, other strategies may be more helpful. One such strategy is called 'paradoxical intention'. This involves doing the opposite of what you want to do. In the case of sleep it involves lying in bed trying not to sleep. If you are just going to lie awake worrying about not sleeping, you may as well try not sleeping – at least you won't be worrying about it! The reasoning behind this is that it takes the force out of the worrying – which is the main thing keeping you awake. Another reason is that it is extremely difficult to stay awake after some time, and so you'll eventually go off to sleep despite your efforts not to. In doing this you'll be able to begin to break the link between worrying and sleep.

If you still find you can't sleep and are worried about your insomnia, it is advisable to seek a referral from your

GP to one of the specialist sleep clinics where sleep patterns can be monitored accurately overnight and a complete physiological and psychological assessment of the nature of the sleep problem can be made.

Restoring disrupted sleep patterns

Another even more rigorous measure has been found to work for those who suffer insomnia because some initial disruption to the sleep pattern has become established and difficult to break. Erratic lifestyles of many sorts often bring about this problem. Students studying late into the night for examinations, deliberately keeping themselves awake, then find it difficult to revert back to a more normal sleep pattern once the examinations are over. Caring for a small child or a sick relative can set up erratic sleep patterns. In fact, any sort of crisis that affects our lives can disrupt our normal sleep patterns. Generally, we revert back to our usual sleep pattern once things have run their course. However, sometimes the disrupted sleep pattern takes hold and it's difficult to re-establish our usual sleep pattern. When all other attempts to re-establish a better sleep pattern have failed, people are sometimes advised to set aside a week or so of their lives in order to deal with the problem. They are advised to stay up an extra two or three hours a night, each night of that week, until they reach an acceptable bedtime hour. In other words, the body clock is readjusted. Trying to re-establish a sleep pattern by going to bed earlier each night doesn't work.

GUIDELINES FOR BETTER SLEEP

As you begin to deal with your problem of insomnia, you may find it helpful to check that you are following these guidelines for good sleep.

1 Deal with specific anxieties during the day or early evening and never later on in the evening or in bed.
2 Avoid stimulating foods and drinks in the evening. These include coffee, tea and alcohol.
3 Avoid stimulating activities late at night, including strenuous exercise, work and arguments.
4 Establish a winding-down routine before you go to bed. Spend the last hour before bedtime preparing for sleep, including some relaxation and a warm bath.
5 Make sure your bedroom is a soothing environment.
6 Make sure that noise isn't disturbing your sleep.

CHAPTER 4

Bringing about Change (1): Achieving a More Balanced Lifestyle

Modern life doesn't encourage natural sleep–wake rhythms. We start work at the same time all year round, whether it is dark or light. Commuter travel is uncomfortable and frustrating. Office atmospheres are often fraught and environmentally unhealthy. Lunch may be a quick sandwich. To try and relax we go to noisy pubs or clubs. It's little wonder that our whole physical, mental and emotional systems are out of step with our natural body rhythms.

Busy people need less activity in their schedule, not more. You may have developed the pattern of constantly 'doing' or 'being on the go' so that 'doing nothing' doesn't appear on your daily agenda – and, indeed, may feel quite threatening. However, 'doing nothing' and allowing yourself both the space and time to think, to daydream or simply go for a walk may be just what you need. But please remember: if you're a perfectionist or over-stressed, don't stress yourself even more by setting yourself impossible targets! Make up your mind about the most important changes to make, and make them. As your physical and mental health begins to regain a better balance, further changes often follow naturally.

COPING WITH STRESS

Self-monitoring – keeping a stress diary

The first step in coping with stress is to find out what makes you anxious in the first place. It can be helpful to keep a diary of feelings, thoughts and anxiety symptoms as they happen in your daily life. In this way you can begin to look at the events and situations that cause you stress. To start with, make up a page of three columns. In the first column, note what happened before you felt stressed. In the second, note what happens when you become anxious – how your body reacts, symptoms of anxiety and the thoughts that go through your mind. In the third, note what happens after the event is over – what makes you worse and what makes you feel better. Symptoms of anxiety aren't just symptoms – usually people become anxious for good reasons.

Case study: Sue

When Sue came to the sleep clinic she found it hard to link how her high daytime anxiety levels prevented her from going off to sleep at night. She didn't know why she was anxious; she was only aware of experiencing the symptoms of anxiety such as sweating and palpitations. I encouraged Sue to keep a stress diary in which she recorded what happened before and after she suffered anxiety symptoms. Over a few sessions a pattern emerged which also helped throw more light on why she couldn't sleep at night.

The following entry from Sue's stress diary reveals how her general apprehension about going out was added to by her drinking coffee. After she experienced her symptoms she'd lie down and find relief in sleep. When she woke up she'd feel despondent that she hadn't managed to go out, which then made her feel even more inadequate. Not only did she make her anxiety worse by avoiding the situation; by withdrawing into sleep during the day she prevented herself from sleeping properly at night which further added to her difficulties the next day.

Sue's stress diary

Date and time	What happened before	Symptoms	What happened after
	Need to go out	Heart races	Decide not to go out
	Drink coffee	Hot, sweaty – frightened 'I can't'	Lie down Sleep

By keeping the diary Sue began to see that her anxiety attack was related to thoughts about going out shopping, and was probably not helped by drinking coffee – which is a stimulant, and would have made her anxiety symptoms worse. As she continues to monitor her anxiety, using the diary, some less obvious sources of stress may emerge. If you are unsure what might be causing your anxiety, keeping a simple stress diary may help you find a pattern.

Make a diary of how anxious or tense you are in the day

Make a note in the margin from 0 to 8 of how tense you are. Start to identify the situations when your tension is high. After you've begun to recognize the increase in tension, that's the time to start putting into action techniques to bring tension down.

How to cope with under-arousal of the stress response

Some people have difficulty in sleeping at night because they are just not doing enough with their lives. Rather than being over-stressed, they are not expending enough physical and mental energy during the day to get good sleep at night. Take a look at your daytime activities and see whether you are getting enough physical exercise and mental stimulation.

If you feel unfulfilled, start working out what you could do over the coming month that would be a real challenge. Write a list of possibilities, things that you may have thought of doing but never got round to doing. We sometimes deny ourselves what we really want by telling ourselves it is impossible. Or else we make excuses for ourselves, either because the idea of change is threatening or we've just got into the habit of self-denial.

How we keep anxiety going and make it worse

We need some anxiety to get us going and gear us up for action. It's only when it reaches the stage where it begins to work against us that anxiety itself is something to worry about. The best way to deal with any fear or anxiety is to face up to it. Trying to ignore or avoid it will only make things worse. There are three methods we use that can make our anxiety worse. These are:

- avoidance
- escape
- reassurance

The more we escape and/or avoid events that make us anxious, the longer our anxiety goes on. This can lead us to suffer from mild to full-blown panic attacks – short bouts of intense anxiety – or even to develop phobias about particular events or situations. Like avoidance and escape, reassurance brings down anxiety in the short term. Because anxiety comes down we are relieved. However, because relief is pleasurable this then acts like a reward to our arousal system. In reality our anxiety is kept going. We repeat the same pattern the next time we face a similar situation and feel even more anxious about it. Explore what it is about situations that is making you anxious and try to find better ways of coping with anxiety than avoidance, escape or reassurance.

SIMPLE FIRST-AID TECHNIQUES

Tension control

When we are wound-up and suffering from stress, we need to give our systems a rest so that they can get back to normal and be ready to deal with the next crisis. This isn't a simple task. Just telling someone to 'relax' won't work.

We'll be looking at relaxation techniques in detail later on, but the simplest first-aid remedy is to become aware of your immediate physical symptoms. If you build into your daily life some simple physical tension control exercises, you'll find that over time you'll feel better and have more control over the physical symptoms of anxiety.

Tension control, like any other form of exercise, improves with practice. Stop what you are doing, concentrate on your shoulders, hunch them right up, drop them, circle the shoulder joints with arms hanging freely at your side. How tense is your neck? Drop the head forward on the chest, let it roll round in a circle under its own weight, keeping the shoulders down. Let your spine go and sag in the middle. Now take ten deep breaths, blowing out all the air in a long breath. You'll feel the tightness go.

Now organize the rest of your day, building in at least four spaces when you'll spend at least five minutes to practise tension control. You'll gradually come to notice small increases in tension in yourself rather than just letting it build up. You'll be more effective at whatever you do if you're calm and not in a state of high tension.

Coping with situations that make us anxious

We can also learn to overcome anxiety related to specific situations or events. Make up a list of ten situations that make you anxious. Number them in order, from those that make you feel most anxious to those that make you feel least anxious. Now you can try a technique for gradually dealing with anxiety. First choose the lowest item on your list.

1 Relax
2 Imagine item
3 Stop imagining
4 Relax

First relax. Imagine your feared situation. Keep relaxing and focussing on bringing your tension levels right down. Now stop imagining and relax. Repeat this several times with the same item until imagining the situation doesn't make you feel anxious. Only go on to a more difficult item when you're fully relaxed with the one lower down on your list. Select no more than two new items each session. Rate your anxiety level from 0 to 8.

First-aid technique for over-arousal or strain

There are some 'first-aid' principles which can provide a brief respite to an over-strained system and help to prevent even more damage for the time being. The following technique can be used equally well whether you're a busy housewife or a busy manager – it can be particularly useful prior to a meeting. If you're too wound up your body will be tense, your thoughts racing and jumbled and your judgement will be clouded.

Tell everyone that you're not to be disturbed for ten minutes. Close the door and take the telephone off the hook. Find the most comfortable chair in the room. Stretch fully from head to toe before sitting down. Now sit down and concentrate on the head and neck. Drop the shoulders, lift the head, thus separating the small bones of the spine by lifting the head from the neck, and look straight ahead. You may be aware of a tight 'ball' in the nape of the neck going into the base of the skull. Press it. If it feels tense, the tension needs to be reduced as it is part of the brain system which helps to control blood pressure. It also deals with arousal and with information going to the brain. Breathe slowly and deeply for ten breaths, becoming aware of warmth at the nape of the neck as you do this. After four of these slow, deep breaths begin to sag with every breath you breathe out, sagging further and further down in the chair with every breath, until you feel limp like a rag doll. Stay like that, just limp, for one minute.

In the time you have left sit comfortably and quietly, keeping your shoulders and neck easy and free. Begin to clear the scrabble in the brain. Breathe away quietly and easily. Calm your mind by just focussing on your breathing. Now give yourself two words, one for breathing in and one for breathing out. For example, say 'calm' to yourself as you slowly breathe in and 'rest' or 'peace' as you slowly breathe out all the air from your lungs. Choose words that you personally find helpful. Saying these to yourself will cut out the other thoughts that are trying to crowd your mind. Now say them more and more quietly until you are just aware of the sounds without 'thinking' them. This cuts out the thoughts already cluttering your brain. As the end of the ten minutes approaches, breathe fully and deeply again for eight breaths, aware of how refreshed and alert you now feel in both mind and body.

CALMING DOWN

There are many things which affect how we deal with stress – our past experiences and the patterns of coping we've developed based on these experiences, our tolerance levels of frustration, anxiety and worry, whether we see challenges as exciting or worrying, the social, personal and work problems which make up our daily lives. However, the best way to deal with stress is to prevent it in the first place. Learning to control our stress can help bring this about.

1   Planning your time

One of the most stressful things in life is the feeling that there's never enough time to do things properly. We've become compulsive clock-watchers. Time seems to rule us. For our physical and mental well-being it's essential that we find some way of managing our time rather than letting it control us. If everything is rushed we lose any pleasure which we may have got and are often left with feelings of frustration, anxiety and worry. To avoid this, organization is essential. Keep a diary of such daily events as appointments, meetings, and so on. Work out the amount of preparation you think you need for these and give yourself enough time to prepare, noting in your diary the start of your preparation time. Prioritize the most important things you have to do on any particular day – even the telephone calls – and take into account the time they might take. Don't worry if they're not all ticked off at the end of the day.

2   Give yourself satisfaction

As you complete a set task during the day, stop and cross it off the list and enjoy the sense of achievement. Only then look at the next priority. Don't take away the pleasure of successfully finishing a task by bringing in worry and pressure about the next thing to be done.

3   Be realistic

A little done well is more stress-reducing than a long list of things which you cannot hope to do. Remember that it's the pleasure of achievement and the positive feedback from this which adds to your resources to face stress in the future.

4   Know your concentration span and energy curve

Everyone's energy curve is different. Some people are wide awake with full high energy first thing in the morning. Others reach their peak at midday and others in the evenings. A test of this is to imagine you have an important exam and no time to study for it during the day. Would you rather get up early in the morning or stay up late at night to do it? You'd naturally choose your highest peak with anything that needs concentration. Working with your own energy curve you'll achieve better results in less time. Concentration usually wanders after about 45 minutes so stop, walk round, rest your eyes and flex your muscles, stretch and relax. Then return to the task feeling refreshed. Performance deteriorates after three hours and that's the time to stop for a light snack and a drink to refuel the energy system. At this time try and take a short break by doing something different. For example, if your work is mostly sedentary and mental, try to get some physical exercise. If you can, go for short walk in the fresh air. Even stretching and deep breathing will get the circulation moving freely which will help the flow of blood to the brain and help reduce tiredness. Don't begrudge the time you take for these breaks – remember you'll feel better and work better.

5   Learn to delegate

Try and let others help, both at home and in the office. Try and involve other people more when you make decisions. Remember, people like to feel needed.

6   Food and drink

A healthy, balanced lifestyle includes good nutrition. Food and drink have a direct chemical influence on our bodies, nervous system and moods. Some foods are more stimulating and some more sedative in their own right. Overindulging in junk food, coffee, tea or alcohol – all of which often go with a stressed lifestyle – affects your feelings of physical and mental well-being. As well as over-stimulating the adrenal glands and nervous system, these foods and drinks deplete the body of essential vitamins and minerals.

We often get contradictory messages about what's good for us and what's harmful. If you want advice see a nutritionist, dietician or naturopath about your own individual needs. There are some general guidelines about food and drink which help promote good sleep (see pages 51–54).

7   Say 'No'

Having an action-packed diary may look impressive, but you may be paying the price in anxiety. Look realistically at your commitments before you add any more to them. Do you have enough time for yourself in your diary? Start to build in some time each day when you can be free to sit and think or just sit.

8   Find something in your work to enjoy

However tedious a task is, you'll find that if you take a positive approach to it you'll feel better about it. Go over the day in your mind and find something in it to be pleased about.

9 Take your foot off the accelerator

You don't have to go flat out through the day. Try pacing yourself. Make sure you're not neglecting your own needs and that you are having the right balance between work or activity and rest throughout the day.

10 Try to maintain a balanced system

There are natural rhythms of movement and rest which we have got used to ignoring because of the demands that we feel are made of us. However, it is less stressful to follow these natural rhythms than work against them. You can start to make your own rhythm to fit into your daily life by keeping as good a balance as possible between physical and mental exercise, between work and relaxation and between activity and sleep. When your body is tired, rest it and exercise the mind. When involved with mental effort, take some physical exercise, if only a short walk.

Regular exercise contributes to general health and well-being. It's also better for good sleep than the occasional over-enthusiastic burst. Research shows that those who exercise consistently have more deep, delta sleep than non-exercisers; when deprived of it their delta sleep decreases. This is because exercise tires the body in a very different way from the tiredness we feel when we rush around getting mentally exhausted or the tiredness we feel when we are lethargic, bored and frustrated. Exercise is a way of clearing the body of the stress hormones that keep many people awake, anxious or depressed. It can also help to clear our bodies if we're trying to give up smoking, alcohol or any other kind of drug. Exercise also releases chemicals in the brain which can help lift our moods and some people find that regular jogging or walking helps them come out of depression.

What kind of exercise?

Don't go in for a sudden enthusiastic burst of exercise if you aren't fit. You may find it too much and get disheartened, or find you can't keep up the unreasonable demands you've put on yourself. Rather build up exercise slowly and gently. There are many things that you can adapt in your everyday life that can improve your exercise. Try walking rather than driving, climbing stairs rather than taking lifts. If you usually spend your lunch hour in a pub or canteen try spending 20 or so minutes of that time walking.

   If you aren't keen on exercise, it may suit you better to join a class. Having a regular commitment to a group helps to keep you motivated. It's also a good way of getting to know new people. Find what suits you – tennis, squash and golf are all beneficial – and find something you enjoy. If you're retired, getting enough exercise will help to keep you healthy. If you've let yourself go, build up slowly by adding a bit more every day. If you're regularly stressed, consider taking up a calming form of movement, like yoga, which calms mind and body. Swimming and walking both encourage deep breathing. If you're anxious or depressed, pick a form of exercise that you enjoy which isn't a form of self-punishment and doesn't increase your competitive tendencies. Activities such as aerobics and dancing – either in a formal class or using a radio or tape at home – are good both for exercise and for lifting your mood. Whatever type of exercise you decide on, commit yourself to doing it regularly, build up slowly and enjoy it!

ACHIEVING THE BALANCE

Pleasure time

Most of our activities have a secondary purpose – to earn a living or to keep the family and household going.

However, some activities can be done for their own sake simply because we enjoy them. Many of us spend a lot of our spare time or relaxation time watching other people do things – on television, at the cinema or sports events. How much time do you spend actually 'doing' something enjoyable rather than just 'watching'? Many people have talents that are just neglected or underused. Whether you are over-stressed or not stressed enough, there's probably something that you always wished you'd been able to do or get involved in – music, painting, getting a degree. Maybe it is that unfulfilled part of you that is contributing towards keeping you awake at night.

Towards self-fulfilment

Do you want to develop the more creative side of yourself, or spend more time with family or friends – or maybe less if you're constantly trying to meet their needs? Think about whether you're really doing what you want to do, or do you have some unfulfilled dream that your lifestyle or internal procedures have so far prevented you from fulfilling? If so, what is the first step to take? You could make a start by writing a list of things that you haven't done but would like to do, however extreme or bizarre they may seem. Just let the ideas flow.

When you've written everything that you can think of, look at the list as if it had been written by another person whom you know well and care about. What is really possible? Maybe it's too late to be a pop star or an opera diva, but you could join a singing class or a choir. You don't have to excel in order to enjoy splashing paint about, to enjoy the stimulation and companionship of a creative writing class or the fun of taking part in an amateur theatrical group. If you feel mentally under-stimulated, it's never too late to take up further education, either by joining night classes or by enrolling on adult educational courses. Even if you don't think that you are particularly

clever or creative, or your domestic set-up makes it difficult to get out to classes, skills that engage your mind and
hands can be satisfying and rewarding.

There are often small things which we can do in our
daily lives that change the way we look at and experience
things. A friend of mine goes for a walk every evening and
sets herself the task of trying to notice and observe everything around her on her walk. In this way even though she
takes the same walk every day, each day it's different
because she makes a point of noticing the small changes in
nature and her surroundings. As you go through the day
make a point of noticing what gives you pleasure or lifts
your spirits, however small.

Maybe you'd like a better social life. Try taking the first
step yourself by asking round the people you'd like to see
more. If you're lethargic, exercise may be more useful than
relaxation. On the other hand, if you're stressed and rush-
ing around all the time, a regular period of relaxation or
meditation may be what you need. The idea is to balance
those aspects of your life that are over-used with those that
have become neglected.

CHAPTER 5

Bringing about Change (2): Relaxation and Meditation

The human brain is divided into two with each half having specific functions. Usually the left hemisphere controls the right side of the body and deals with functions like speech and logical thinking. The right hemisphere, which controls the left side of the body, is responsible for abstract thought, dreaming, intuition and visual imagery. In our work-oriented world most people use the logical side most of the time at the expense of the right. It's this intuitive side of the brain that's responsible for producing many insights and solutions to problems that our reason and logic alone have been unable to solve. When we allow more right-hemisphere activity the brain waves slow down from the active beta rate to the alpha rhythm that usually precedes sleep. We then become more peaceful and more creative. This state of mind can be achieved through relaxation and meditation and also through the use of mental imagery and visualization. These techniques can help restore harmony to daytime life as well as enable us to sleep better at night.

RELAXATION

Some people find it difficult to relax simply because they don't know what relaxation feels like. Many natural therapies can help you to regain that experience, particularly physical treatments like massage. Some forms of exercise are also very relaxing. Yoga includes techniques for whole body relaxation and meditation, while some forms of martial arts such as T'ai Chi have been described as meditation in movement.

Regular relaxation can actually alter body chemistry, and deep states can help the brain to produce endorphins which have the effect of lifting the mood and relieving pain. Meditation has many similar effects. Although relaxation is aimed mainly at the body and meditation at the mind, both slow down and rebalance the body–mind system. Many people who meditate regularly find they need less sleep than before because during their meditation periods they are giving their systems deep rest. Both meditation and relaxation require us – and enable us – to let go of worry and tension and focus on the present moment.

Some people are quite frightened of letting go. They feel they have to stay in control. And yet letting go is a normal part of life's rhythm. Hanging on to control builds up physical tensions which you take to bed with you. A tense mind is less able to solve problems than a relaxed one. If you learn to relax you'll find that you'll have more control over your waking and sleeping patterns. Most people could benefit from regular relaxation or meditation. Build it into your day.

Learning to relax

You can join a class where you can learn relaxation or you can carry it out on your own. If you want to do it on your own try and set aside a time each day, maybe 20 minutes or so, to carry out a simple relaxation exercise. Often when we are busy and anxious we feel that we don't have time to relax, but think about this. In a way we seem to be saying that we're too tense to learn to relax. But by learning to relax you can become more aware of the build-up of tension and learn to do something about it. With practice, you'll begin to notice the early stages of tension in your body, and you can learn to control it at this early stage instead of letting the tension increase.

To learn to relax first find a quiet room where you'll be peaceful and undisturbed. Devote 20 minutes to completely letting go. Sit comfortably with your back supported and your feet flat on the floor, your hands loose in your lap and your eyes closed. Or lie down with your head and knees supported by cushions. You can listen to a cassette – there are many relaxation tapes on the market – or you can record your own version. You can start to learn to relax your muscles without even using a tape. There are several relaxation techniques to help better sleep. Here are three.

Relaxation exercise 1

Progressive relaxation consists of going through your whole body tensing and relaxing each part in turn, from the feet working right up to the forehead, breathing slowly and evenly until you've let go of all tensions and feel relaxed and calm. First of all, close your eyes and try to relax to the best of your ability. Begin by taking in six deep breaths, hold each breath for a count of 3, and then release all the air from your lungs. It's important not to breathe in more than you breathe out, otherwise you may feel light-headed and dizzy due to over-breathing.

1 Close your eyes and let your whole body relax. Breathe in and out slowly and evenly.
2 Hands. Start with your left hand. Tighten your fist, feel the tension, then let it go, let the muscles slacken and relax the hand. Work up to your left forearm and upper arm, and then proceed with your right fist, forearm and upper arm. Concentrate on getting rid of all the tension in your hands and arms. Even when they feel

completely relaxed, try to relax them a little bit more. Try to achieve deeper and deeper levels of relaxation. Now do the same for each part of the body in turn as follows.

3 Shoulders.
4 Neck and throat.
5 Face, forehead, eyes, jaws and mouth.
6 Chest.
7 Back.
8 Stomach.
9 Bottom and thighs.
10 Legs, shins, calves, ankles.
11 Feet.

Your whole body should now feel quite relaxed. See if you can feel any tension anywhere in your body and concentrate on getting rid of it. Let your whole body relax, enjoy the feeling of relaxation and continue like that for a few minutes. You can then become even more relaxed by taking in a really deep breath and slowly breathing out. Just continue relaxing like that for a few minutes more. Enjoy the sense of relaxation until your 20 minutes are up. Come out of it slowly. If you get up too quickly you may find yourself feeling slightly giddy.

Like everything else, to relax well you need practice. If you've been tense over a long period of time, it will take time for your body to learn how to let go of the tension. It is a good idea to practise the relaxation routine daily to begin with.

Relaxation exercise 2

Once your body has been tuned in to the above relaxation exercise you can fit this shortened version into your everyday life, using it whenever you feel the need to relax.

Choose a comfortable seat or lean against something. If you don't wish to go through all of the above exercise you can choose a few body parts which feel tense, such as the neck or calf muscles, and use the same tensing and let-ting-go relaxation procedure. Breathe in a normal size breath to a count of 3, hold it for a count of 3 and then breathe out slowly, releasing tension as you do so. Say to yourself 'relax' as you breathe out. Do this twice. Now go back to breathing at your own natural pace, calmly and evenly.

Relaxation exercise 3

Another method is to start sitting or lying, stretch the whole body and let it go like a cat. Then simply study the relax-ation throughout your body as you breathe slowly in and out, while more and more tension is leaving you with every out-breath.

Relaxation can be helped by using mental imagery. As you let go physically, imagine that you're floating on a cloud or a balloon in the sky or lying on a warm beach. Images of both lightness and heaviness seem to help relax-ation equally well. Find the one that best suits you. What you're aiming for is the ability to relax whenever you want to – not just at special relaxation times.

MEDITATION

Meditation takes you into a relaxed state through the mind. The aim is to reach a state of inner peace by qui-etening thoughts, often by focussing on a word, sound or object. People find it useful to join a class as beginners often strain to concentrate and guidance may be helpful in learning to let go. If you want to try it for yourself, start with five or ten minutes at a time. Sit as for the relaxation exercise above. Make sure you won't be disturbed, then try the following example.

Meditation exercise

Gently repeat mentally a single word, for example 'calm'. Rest your attention on this word without straining. Every time you find your mind wandering, bring it back to the word.

Pay attention to your breathing. Simply be aware of it without trying to change it. It can help you to concentrate if you count slowly from one to ten – 'one and', 'two and' and so on – with each in–out breath.

At the end of any relaxation or meditation, don't leap back into activity, but come out slowly and gently, bringing some of that feeling of inner calm into the rest of your life.

BREATHING

Correct breathing is important in both relaxation and meditation. As body and mind slow down so does the breath. Slowing and deepening your breathing automatically makes you calmer. However, when we're tense we tend to breathe fast and shallow, high up in the chest. This makes it very difficult to relax. Some habitually tense people hyperventilate. This means they overbreathe all the time, which keeps them in a permanent state of anxiety. Hyperventilation can have other unpleasant side-effects like migraines, dizziness, nausea and palpitations.

Learning to breathe naturally helps you to keep calm. Try the following exercise.

Breathing exercise 1

Lie on the floor with a cushion or book under your head. Put an object such as a large book on your midriff, between your stomach and lower ribs. As you breathe in and out, the object should rise and fall. If it doesn't, you're breathing too high up in your chest. Using the weight as a guide, you can retrain yourself to breathe from the diaphragm. Full breathing should expand your diaphragm, lower ribs and stomach. Don't force yourself to breathe deeply. Just be aware of how you're breathing at the moment. Think of your ribs and lungs expanding and contracting and allow your breath to become deeper, slower and calmer. Think of your ribs expanding sideways as well as up and down. If you practise this for a few minutes every day, you'll get used to breathing in a calmer, more relaxing way when you go to bed at night.

Breathing exercise 2

A symptom of anxiety is holding your breath. A good exercise when you feel yourself tensing up during the day is to consciously breathe out, at the same time letting the tension flow away from your neck, shoulders and arms. Practise this in situations which would usually make you tense – for example, lining up, in traffic hold-ups, waiting. You can use these situations as opportunities to try out relaxation instead of anxiety, frustration or anger and irritation.

VISUALIZATION

The imagination can have a direct effect on our body, for good or ill. For example, when you mentally recall a traumatic incident that has happened in your life, your heart can start racing, your pulse quicken and your breathing become more shallow as the body's stress system gets into action. It doesn't matter that the incident isn't real. Your body and nervous system react as though it is. Similarly, when you imagine pleasant or happy experiences your body relaxes and you're mentally more peaceful. Alternative therapists often use visualization to help their own healing process. When you start imagining yourself healthy and happy your body starts to feel healthier and stronger. In a relaxed, daydreaming state you can mentally picture any outcome that you want, whether it's better sleep or carrying out some task. It's important to believe and expect that what you visualize will come about as in this way you affect your expectations which then influence behaviour.

Visualization techniques may not be right for everyone. If you're an anxious achiever, you may put too much effort into what should be effortless or even make yourself worse by focussing on symptoms rather than health. Even if you don't use specific techniques, you naturally use the power of thought and imagination throughout the day, both mentally and visually. You can actually replace depressing thoughts about your life and your sleep with positive ideas about what you really want.

The first essential step for visualization is to be able to relax deeply. If you're normally tense, you may need quite a lot of practice in learning to relax.

Visualization exercise – 'descending lift' method of deepening relaxation

You can record this for yourself, pausing in the appropriate places, and play it back while you are sitting comfortably or lying down in a relaxed position, perhaps even in bed before going to sleep.

Imagine that you are standing on the fifth floor of a large department store … You are just stepping into the lift … to go down to street level. And as you go down … the lift doors open and close at each floor … and you will become more and more relaxed … and your sleep will become deeper and deeper. The lift doors are closing now … and you are beginning to sink slowly downwards … The lift stops at the fourth floor … several people get out … two more get in … the doors close again … and already you are becoming more and more deeply relaxed … more and more deeply asleep. And as you sink to the third floor ... and stop, while the doors open and close again ... you are relaxing more and more ... and your sleep becomes deeper and deeper. You slowly sink to the second floor ... one or two people get out and several get in ... and as they do so ... you are feeling much more deeply relaxed ... much more deeply asleep. Down you go again to the first floor ... the doors open and close ... but nobody gets out or in. Already you have become still more deeply relaxed ... and your sleep deeper and deeper. Deeper and deeper asleep, deeper and deeper asleep. Down further and further ... until at last the lift stops at street level ... The doors open ... and everybody gets out ... but you do not get out ... you decide to go still deeper ... descending to the basement. The lift doors close again ... and down you go ... down and down ... deeper and deeper ... and as you arrive at the basement ... you are feeling twice as deeply and comfortably relaxed ... twice as deeply asleep.

Visualization exercise – calming your nightmares

Sometimes our dreams disturb us and wake us up at night. If these happen frequently and are very frightening, you may need to seek help from a professional counsellor or therapist. However, many people find that they can help themselves gain some control over their nightmares and reduce their fear of them by adapting a traditional technique used by the native American Navajo to change the content of their nightmares. You can do this by first carrying out a relaxation exercise.

When you're fully relaxed and sitting or lying down calmly and peacefully with your eyes shut, start going through your nightmare. When you reach a frightening bit, try and remain as physically and mentally relaxed as possible and change the frightening part into something that you feel comfortable with. Make sure you're fully relaxed and calm before going through the nightmare again and repeating the exercise. If it's the ending of the nightmare that frightens you – it's usually the part that wakes you up – change the ending. If you experience the nightmare during the night, go into another room and carry out the exercise, returning to bed only when you feel relaxed and calm. You can practise this as part of your relaxation routine during the day. In this way you gain more control over your nightmare and fears.

CHAPTER 6

Bringing About Change (3): Learning Better Ways of Coping with our Emotions

We all have patterns of thinking, behaving and feeling that are very much part of ourselves and the way that we deal with ourselves, our relationships and the world in general. Many of these patterns began very early on in our lives as we developed ways of coping with our experiences. Together they form the belief systems – our beliefs, thoughts and assumptions – that govern our behaviour towards ourselves and others. However, what worked earlier on may no longer be effective. It may even work against us.

Whether you feel anxious, depressed or unfulfilled, or have a particular problem that you've been worrying about or putting off dealing with, it's important to start the process of change. The more you put off doing something about an unsatisfactory situation the worse it's likely to get and the more your mind will churn over your problems when you try to go to sleep at night. Most of us can learn to feel better about ourselves, just as we can learn any new skill. But you'll have to take the first step, by making the decision to change.

Changing means looking at our fears and anxieties – however large or small they may be – and the faulty thinking, ideas and beliefs that often lie behind them and hold them in place. It also means having the courage to react differently – for example, being able to say 'no' without fearing we are letting others down. Change doesn't have to be dramatic. It may be just a change in one thought, but a small change can be enough to start a knock-on effect that spreads throughout the rest of our experiences.

The following are guidelines which you may find useful to follow to help you begin the process of change.

- Writing your life story.
- Gathering information.
- Naming the problem.
- Learning to express your feelings.

WRITING YOUR LIFE STORY

By writing down your life story – what happened to you and how things have come to be as they are in your life – you'll begin to look at what it is you need or wish to change.

1 You can begin by describing your own family, your early experiences and your feelings about people and events when you were a child. Then go on systematically through your life, dating significant events and how you felt about yourself and others in your life at those points. Some people find it easier to write their life story in the third person, as though a close friend who knows them well and cares about them were writing it.

2 When you feel you have all the important experiences and facts you'd like, take a good look at what you've written. Begin to notice what effect your early experiences and your attitude to them has had on the way you think and feel about yourself and others and on the way you act in the world now.

3 End your story by writing something about the changes you'd like to make and how you might begin making them. These can be changes in the way you think about yourself, faulty thinking patterns and false beliefs. Or they may be changes in particular patterns such as pleasing others, negative thinking or avoidance.

Writing our life story can be an enlightening experience, and when we view our story with compassion and kindness a very moving one. Through this process we can begin to see how our life has been, how the attitudes we formed early on to ourselves and others have contributed to the difficulties we have, and how by changing these attitudes we can start to move away from what we may have believed to be fixed characteristics or unchangeable habits over which we had no control. It may even be the first time we realize that we can have some control over our life. Writing our story also helps to sort out confusion and give us greater clarity of how things are and how they've been rather than just muddling along hoping that somehow fate will deal us a better hand.

GATHERING INFORMATION

Self-monitoring

The main purpose of self-monitoring is to increase your awareness of your own patterns. With increased awareness you can become quicker at spotting how one thing leads to another in terms of your own and other people's reactions. Once you understand the process and how it operates, you have a chance to stop or change the process.

What do you monitor? You can monitor any of your feelings, thoughts and ways of coping and behaving which cause you distress or may be symptoms of your distress. For example, you may wish to monitor physical symptoms such as headaches, forgetfulness, symptoms of stress and anxiety. You may monitor your feelings, such as depression and unhappiness. You can also monitor thoughts about yourself and others or behaviour such as smoking, eating, sleeping.

Carry a small notebook around with you that you can look at easily. When you make an entry write down the time of day, place, who else is around, what else is happening and, most important, what you're thinking and feeling at the time. Keep this notebook for a week before studying it. Sometimes we have to keep up the monitoring for a few weeks before we can see any kind of pattern.

When you read through the entries in your notebook pick out one or more themes or phrases that come up regularly, noting the time and place and who else was present. It was through self-monitoring in this way that one woman learned that her headaches were worse when she was unable to stand up for herself. It was as though the headache acted as a reminder that she needed to express herself more and not just passively accept everything without comment.

NAMING THE PROBLEM

1 Learn to recognize your beliefs

The fact is that every one of us, to some degree, holds some negative beliefs about ourselves and the world. The important thing to realize is that, although they may seem to be true to us, they are only beliefs and have no objective truth.

As you read through these negative thoughts and ideas, see whether any of them apply to your own belief system or are the underlying assumptions which are reflected in the ways you feel or behave.

There's something wrong with me.
I'm worthless and don't deserve anything good.

I've done things (or a bad thing) in my life and I deserve to suffer or be punished for it.

People (including me) are basically bad – selfish, cruel, stupid, untrustworthy, foolish, etc.

The world is an unsafe place.

Life is painful, suffering, hard work . . . it's not meant to be fun.

Getting involved with anyone is dangerous . . . I might get hurt.

Power is dangerous . . . I might hurt someone.

I don't have control over what happens to me . . . I'm powerless to do anything about my life or the state of the world.

2   Learning to recognize your thoughts

i   The way we think about ourselves and our lives influences the way that we feel about ourselves

Even though patterns of thinking may seem to us natural and inevitable, if you take a close look at your pattern of thinking you may well find that the pattern could be working against you. The way that we think about ourselves is often the result of what we've been told about ourselves, both now and in the past, by people whose opinions matter to us, such as parents, family and friends.

Case study: Luke

Luke had always been seen by his family as 'lazy'. He'd always put things off and seemed unable to make decisions. He'd always got by at school by being the comic of the class and he was still always the first to laugh at his own mistakes. He'd always been likable and popular and often found people who were happy to help him out. However, when the time came that he had to face serious difficulties in his life he just couldn't believe he could deal with them so he didn't try. Gradually things mounted up and he became more and more stressed, suffering from symptoms of anxiety during the day and from difficulty in getting to sleep at night. Eventually, as things went from bad to worse, he saw his family doctor who at first prescribed tranquillizers to help him to cope better during the day and sleep at night. Luke found that after a while he needed more tablets to calm him down and went back to his doctor who referred him for therapy. It was during therapy that Luke started questioning whether he was as helpless as he'd thought he was and whether, in fact, he really was just 'the lazy one of the family'.

Often we're not aware that we're thinking negatively, thinking in fixed, unproductive ways or making mountains out of molehills. If we tell ourselves all the time 'I can't do it' then we are always setting up expectations that we'll fail, and won't even try to do things. This tends to be a vicious circle in which we end up feeling useless and incapable of doing things.

Experiment by picking out some of your unhelpful thoughts. For example, if you can identify a negative thought such as 'I can't do it' you can try replacing it with a positive thought such as 'I can have a go – nothing really terrible is likely to happen'.

ii *Changing your self-talk – the running commentary*

If you really pay attention to your thoughts then you can know what they are and they can be changed. You can see if your anxiety is based on reality or is based on old or faulty ways of thinking. One technique for finding out more about how you think and how these are linked to how you feel is to make a running commentary on yourself. This process is one in which you are your own observer. Start by asking yourself questions such as 'What do I feel like when . . . ?' Note your thoughts and symptoms as your tension increases. Comment on what happens to your body when tension increases – just like a sports commentator to yourself.

iii Catastrophizing

Suppose you don't get that report done, pass that exam, get that job, clean the house from top to bottom before your parents arrive, and so on – is it really a matter of life or death? Do we really need to put our stress response in top gear? If you're stressed about any event that is looming take a moment and ask yourself, 'What is the worst that can happen if I don't finish the task or achieve the result I want?' Would it really be the end of the world or the catastrophe that you've geared up your stress response to face? Try asking yourself, 'What if such and such a situation happened?' and giving more realistic replies. Look back at the last time when you worried and worried about something. Did it really turn out as badly as you feared? Probably not.

LEARNING TO EXPRESS YOUR FEELINGS

Learning not to bottle up your feelings

Keep some paper on which to write you daily thoughts and ideas. In this way you're keeping a record of what you're feeling and experiencing, what kind of thoughts you're having, what's happening to you. You may like to keep your diary every day or just for when you feel things strongly. Some people prefer to write poems or draw, doodle or paint. Express yourself in the form which comes easier to you. Whatever it is, put it in your diary. The important thing is the meaning it has for you.

Feelings, of course, can be pleasant as well as unpleasant. Try not to 'bottle them up'. The best way to deal with them is to try and become more aware of your feelings and if possible try and express them. Trustworthy friends and family members may be able to help you discover or express these feelings. However, if these feelings seem too confusing or overwhelming, it might be best to consult your doctor. The doctor might well refer you for counselling or psychotherapy to a qualified professional. Or if your problems are specific, such as particular fears and phobias, there may be self-help groups in your area.

Sadness and depression

We all get unhappy and sad from time to time and this can affect our sleep at night. Feelings of sadness, discouragement, unhappiness and disappointment are perfectly normal during difficult, stressful times and especially when we're experiencing unhappy life events such as bereavement, redundancy or divorce. Depression is the most common of all mental health problems and comes in many forms and degrees of severity. If your depression is severe or has gone on for some time then it's a good idea to see your family doctor and seek professional help.

Depressed people are usually very self-critical – you are such as dreadful person you don't deserve to be happy. However, it really is possible to tackle this by beginning to challenge your ways of thinking. As we saw in the last chapter, your usual way of thinking seems natural and automatic to you. Start listening to your self-talk and ask yourself whether you'd be as hard on anyone else.

Life events such as death, divorce, moving house and changing jobs are all stressful events. If your depression is due to life circumstances, such as unemployment, loneliness or financial difficulties, it is perfectly understandable and natural to feel unhappy. Some things are out of our control and we simply cannot change them. Rather than railing against fate or beating your head against a brick wall, try working towards some sort of acceptance of these events. Write down the aspects of your life that are making you unhappy. Look at the list and decide what can be changed. Also consider whether you can get together with other people in the same boat to support each other or join a self-help group. You may find that any effort, however small, will make you feel a bit better.

Many older people are often depressed because they feel lonely and useless. Family and friends move away or die and it can feel as though nobody cares. However, that may be because nobody knows. You may have to make the first move. Old age in itself doesn't have to mean mental deterioration. Make sure that you have a regular routine, giving yourself proper meals and whatever exercise you can. Even if your body is slowing down, look for outside activities that can provide company and mental stimulation.

Be assertive

When we're revising our old patterns of thinking and behaving we often need to be more assertive about our needs and wishes. But we can easily confuse assertion with aggression and hold back from expressing ourselves. If it's difficult for us to be assertive, it may mean that we're afraid that if we express ourselves we'll be too aggressive and hurt others or be seen as too pushy. Yet if we avoid being assertive because of this belief, others may tend to ignore us or take us for granted because they actually don't know what we think or feel. Holding back can also stop us from facing up to the challenge of change. Being assertive is appropriate and acceptable. Learning how to be assertive may be an important part of your changing.

Anger and resentment

Uncomfortable emotions such as anger and resentment are common causes of night-time worry and brooding. If you're angry about a current situation, either accept it or do something about it otherwise all the negative energy and stress will go on keeping you awake. Many people fear confrontations but it is possible to say what you feel about a situation without having a violent explosion. Telling the person or people concerned calmly how you feel about their behaviour without blaming or accusing them can often open up communications so that the problem may be discussed and sorted out. Stick to describing your own thoughts and feelings rather than blaming the other person. This will only result in them defending their position.

If you can't speak to the other person directly, or if the situation which is making you angry happened in the past, tell yourself that whatever anybody else has said or done it's now over. Keeping hold of it is only hurting you. While you're brooding, going over the scene, rehearsing the remarks you could have made or intend to make, the other person may well have forgotten the whole event. The only person who's making you angry now is you, every time you mentally relive these scenes. When you're angry, muscles tense, giving rise to headaches and muscle pain as well as triggering the release of stress hormones all of which can contribute to your insomnia. Keeping hold of anger not only keeps you awake but can lead to physical problems. High blood pressure, heart problems and arthritis are sometimes said to be effects of long-harboured anger.

Try and get anger and resentment out of your system during the day. Although this isn't easy, once you realize that they are only harming you, you can at least decide to let them go.

Dealing with anger and resentment: exercise 1

One way to get short-term relief from anger which is stopping your sleep is the pillow-bashing technique. Find a time and place where you can be alone and make the pillow the focus of your anger. Thump it and shout at the same time. Let go and keep shouting and thumping until you're exhausted, feel drained of your angry feelings and your shoulders and arms have released all that tension.

You can find ways which work for you. Some people find that going for a drive and shouting at the top of their voice works. Other people find that writing a letter to the person about whom they feel angry and then tearing it up works best for them.

Dealing with anger and resentment: exercise 2

Visualization techniques can be helpful in dealing with anger and resentment. In a relaxed state you can visualize the other person – imagine a conversation in which you are feeling differently towards them. Many depressed people suffer from guilt and anger towards themselves. Use visualization to let go of those feelings, reminding yourself of all the good things about yourself.

Resentment and hostility: forgiveness

We often carry the negative feelings of resentment and hostility with us long after the events or people concerned have gone from our lives. The only person these feelings harm is ourselves. Many religions stress the power of prayer in forgiving our enemies. Whether religious or not, many people find that having positive thoughts about past hurts is an effective way of dealing with them. Below is one technique for doing this which you may wish to try out.

Write down on a piece of paper a list of names of everyone in your life who you feel has ever mistreated you, harmed you, done you an injustice or towards whom you feel or have felt resentment, hurt or anger. Next to each person's name write down what they did to you, or what you resent them for.

Then close your eyes, relax and one by one visualize or imagine each person. Hold a conversation with each one and explain to him or her that in the past you have felt anger or hurt towards them, but that now you are going to do your best to forgive them. Many people find that this process of forgiveness relieves them of resentment and hostility.

Now write down the names of everyone you can think of in your life whom you feel you have hurt or done an injustice and write down what you did to them. Again close your eyes, relax and imagine each person in turn. Tell them what you did and ask them to forgive you. Then picture them doing the same and forgiving you.

RELATIONSHIPS AND SLEEP PROBLEMS

You can't change other people: you can only change how you feel and your reactions to them. But what you can do is to tell them how you feel. Don't presume that they know how you feel – people can't read minds. Give them the chance to tell you how they feel. People often make totally false assumptions about what's going on in someone else's mind. Talk openly and honestly. Listening to the other person's point of view as well as expressing your own can clarify a situation.

Marital problems

Most marriages and partnerships go through bad patches, and feeling angry and resentful towards your partner can be a major source of sleeplessness. Do try to resolve your problems during the day or early evening. Don't leave it until bedtime to have rows. Don't lie in bed brooding over your partner's faults and telling yourself that if only he or she were different you'd be happy. Sex is one activity that's good to carry out in bed and doesn't lead to insomnia – the assumption being that you then drop off to sleep happy and relaxed. However, an unsatisfactory sexual relationship can leave one partner feeling worse off than with no sex at all. As with all other problems causing insomnia, it's important to do something about it. The longer difficulties build up the more difficult they can be to solve. Sometimes when couples have difficulties it may be helpful to have a regular weekly date and time for expressing their wishes and grievances in turn, and listening to each other without interruption.

Women and anger

Women often have difficulty in acknowledging that they are angry at all. The idea is often instilled in us from childhood that anger isn't very nice and other people – especially men – will reject us if we're angry. There's some truth in this. Psychological studies show that when men behave in a certain way it's called 'assertive' and 'manly', and is admired. In women the same behaviour is called 'aggressive' and we are put down with derogatory terms such as 'shrew' or 'bitch'. Some women put aside their own wishes and needs in order to be perfect wives and mothers for others. They don't realize that they're angry at always being a doormat and resentful at not having their own needs met. This can lead to a build-up of resentment and anger and trigger off insomnia.

If you need more help to help clarify your feelings and deal with problems in your relationship, consult a marriage guidance counsellor. It is often the confused feelings to do with relationships that can keep us awake at night.

LIVING IN THE PRESENT

Living in the present helps us to accept ourselves as we are without judging ourselves by other people's standards. However, like everything else, this takes practice and may not come easily at first. Once you've got into the habit of living in the present you can try doing the same thing at bedtime. Instead of worrying about if or when you're going to sleep, just try being in the present moment, without going over past regrets or worrying about the future. Try giving your body and mind permission to let go and rest.

Try living in the present as much as you can. Try out the following exercise.

Pay complete attention to whatever you're doing at the time you're doing it, whatever the activity – working, walking or reading. Try focussing on the moment. Be aware of your physical body, your physical surroundings. If you are out walking, try making a point of observing everything – sights and sounds. Gradually you'll become practised in learning to switch off the over-active mind and give both it and you a break.

OTHER WAYS OF HELPING US CHANGE

Finding professional help

Friends and partners can be a great support during the process of change, but sometimes people who know you well will try to cheer you up or change the subject when what would be more helpful is for someone to listen sympathetically. Sometimes they themselves may be part of the cause of your problems and you'll find it difficult to tell them what's on your mind. Getting help in order to help yourself is a much healthier way forward than staying stuck.

Some people feel embarrassed or ashamed at seeking help from a professional such as a psychotherapist or counsellor, yet many personal problems can be helped by short-term counselling. For example, psychotherapy can be helpful in unravelling childhood events and early relationships that are a source of many of our present ways of thinking, feeling and behaving. A good counsellor or therapist will accept who you are and listen to you in a way that friends and family may not be able to.

Formal counselling isn't always necessary. Often it's the qualities of the therapist which are the main factor, whether or not they've been formally trained in counselling. At other times the caring attention and even the touch of a natural practitioner such as a massage therapist, aromatherapist, osteopath or other such healers may gently encourage relaxation and relieve the stresses and strains built up in the body and without the need for in-depth emotional exploration.

CHAPTER 7

Natural Therapies and the Treatment of Insomnia

The range of natural therapies which can be effective in the treatment of insomnia include acupuncture, the Alexander technique, aromatherapy, Bach flower remedies, homeopathy, kinesiology, massage, medical herbalism, the metamorphic technique, natural reconnective therapy, naturopathy, osteopathy and chiropractic (also cranial osteopathy or cranio-sacral therapy), reflexology, reflex zone therapy, shiatsu and spiritual healing.

Natural therapies emphasize that we all have the power and ability to heal ourselves. Rather than treating the symptoms of physical and mental ill-health with a variety of drugs, natural therapies try to remove the obstacles to health and self-healing by restoring balance. The methods and techniques of natural therapies vary. However, they work on the principle that the body, mind and emotions are one interdependent unit. All three elements have to be in balance in order to achieve good health. Therapies which deal with the whole person in this way are called 'holistic'.

As well as relieving medical problems, natural therapies can alleviate pain and help those suffering from insomnia by aiding relaxation and reducing emotional stress and physical tension. Treatment methods used in natural therapy range from direct contact – for example, osteopathy, chiropractic, aromatherapy and massage – to the more indirect methods, which use medication, such as homeopathy or medical herbalism. Many natural therapy practitioners also use counselling to give patients help and support in dealing with the causes of insomnia or with withdrawal from sleeping tablets.

There are a large number of natural therapies generally available. Some of these are complementary to what is termed orthodox medicine while others are viewed as alternative therapies. Natural therapies differ from orthodox medicine in two main ways:

1 Natural therapies treat the whole person rather than that part of the person which is called 'the disease'. They take into consideration the patient's characteristics and lifestyle, and recognize that people vary in their responses to the same treatment.
2 The speed with which treatments are expected to work also differs. For example, antibiotics are increasingly prescribed in orthodox medicine and a course of treatment is relatively quick. However, antibiotics work by suppressing symptoms. In natural medicine symptoms are regarded as the body's efforts to defend itself and treatment consists of strengthening the mind and body which have become depleted enough for harmful bacteria and viruses to flourish. As natural therapies deal with the whole person, not just the symptoms, treatment can take longer to have effect – often months rather than days or weeks. Fortunately, as natural therapies are often very relaxing in themselves, insomnia is often one of the first symptoms to disappear.

The methods of diagnosis are also very different from those used in orthodox medicine. For example, some therapists are trained in iridology, which is diagnosis through the iris of the eye which reflects the state of the body. By this method, variations in the eye such as colour can point to organic or functional weaknesses and nutritional deficiencies. Others use kinesiology techniques to test imbalances and nutritional needs, while other may use techniques such as dowsing with a pendulum.

If you're already on prescribed medication you should discuss this with both your family doctor and alternative or natural practitioner. Some forms of natural medicine are alternative rather than complementary to conventional medicine. For example, many herbal medicines may not be compatible with medical drugs while the effect of some homeopathic remedies can be counteracted by drugs. You should talk to your doctor before making any changes or additions to what he or she has already prescribed for you.

FINDING A NATURAL PRACTITIONER

The number of natural therapies available can be confusing, especially if you don't know much about them and are wondering which one to choose. Sometimes within one particular type of therapy, there are even a number of different training schools which vary in both their approach and emphasis. What is important, however, is that you find the therapy and therapist that are right for you. Often the individual qualities of the therapist are the crucial factor in effective therapy rather than a particular technique or approach.

A frequent way to find a good practitioner is by personal recommendation. Some family doctors have contacts with non-medical practitioners who they recommend to their patients. Another way is to go to a holistic or natural health clinic where a number of different practitioners are available. There someone should advise you as to the most appropriate therapy for you. Some clinics are run in collaboration with medically trained doctors who can give medical advice if necessary. Going to a clinic also means that you can be referred to different practitioners if necessary, all based in the same place.

Before starting a course of treatment it is important to check out the training and range of expertise of the practitioner. Some have trained in more than one therapy and can combine different treatments. Like all other therapies, natural therapies have tightened up their qualifications and regulations. If you choose a practitioner from a newspaper make sure they are properly qualified and belong to a professional register.

ACUPUNCTURE

This ancient Chinese technique is based on the theory that health depends on a harmonious flow of energy, or life force, called *qi* (pronounced chee). *Qi* flows through the body via energy channels – called meridians – of which there are 12. Each of the twelve meridians is connected to and named after a physical organ – the heart, lungs, liver, kidneys, and so on – each of which can be affected by a specific emotion. For example, fear affects the kidneys and anger the liver, together with their relevant meridians. Insomnia is usually found to relate to a disruption in the energy flow of the heart meridian. In traditional Chinese terms the heart is said to be the seat of the mind or spirit and, according to this view, sleeplessness is caused by a turbulent spirit. In more orthodox terms, treating the heart meridian takes the pressure off the nerves to the heart, which may be over-stimulated.

Too much or too little energy in one or more meridians can give rise to both mental and physical symptoms. In acupuncture the diagnosis focusses on the person's state of energy rather than on specific diseases. Traditional methods include taking a full history, observing the patient's skin colour and noting which parts of the body are more hot or cold. The strength of the meridians is checked through 12 pulses found in the wrists. Over- or under-activity in a meridian can be caused by dietary, physical or emotional factors – often a combination of these – and the acupuncturist's aim is to restore health by restoring the balance. The progress of recovery in acupuncture is usually slow and steady.

Along the meridians lie hundreds of acupuncture points, tiny gateways into the energy flow, whose Chinese names often indicate their function. Treatment consists of stimulating or sedating the meridians to restore the energy balance by inserting very fine steel needles into the appropriate points. Whether this is experienced as painful or not depends both on the practitioner's touch and also the patient's sensitivity. Points that need treatment are usually tender to the touch and may be slightly painful when the needle is first inserted. As the balance is restored the pain lessens. Usually only a few points are treated in any one session. The needles may be left in place for 10 to 20 minutes and the acupuncturist may twiddle them around from time to time. Some practitioners treat the acupuncture points with burning herbs rather than needles. For insomnia the acupuncturist may well treat points on the heart meridian.

Acupuncture can be an effective treatment for insomnia, restoring balance and harmony to the patient's energy system. Although many people report they can feel very relaxed even after one treatment session, most people find that overcoming insomnia and establishing better sleep may take several sessions. Practitioners point out that acupuncture can relieve emotional as well as physical pain, reduce anxiety and lift depression. Although many orthodox medical practitioners had reservations about this treatment in the past, it is now the most widely used complementary therapy within the medical profession and is practised by a growing number of family doctors as well as being increasingly used in hospital pain relief clinics.

Acupuncture can also be extremely useful in reducing withdrawal symptoms from tranquillizers, sleeping pills and other drugs including nicotine. Some research findings suggest that acupuncture increases the brain's output of endorphins which reduces pain and lifts the mood. It also helps the body get rid drugs from the system. Some acupuncturists prefer patients to come off their pills before starting any treatment as the drugs may work against the effects of acupuncture.

THE ALEXANDER TECHNIQUE

The Alexander technique was developed over 90 years ago by an Australian actor, Frederick Matthias Alexander. Specializing in one-man shows, he suffered from recurrent hoarseness and breathing problems which prevented him from performing on stage. When medical specialists could find nothing wrong with his throat, Alexander decided that there must be something wrong with the way he was using it. He studied himself with the help of mirrors and realized that his voice was being affected by the way he held his head and neck, which in turn related to the tensions in his body. Over the years he taught himself new habits, not only solving his voice problem but discovering a new mental power and energy.

Advocates of the Alexander technique point out that children from an early age know how to hold themselves. However, they are soon thrown out of balance from schooldays onwards by things such as badly designed school desks and too much time spent sitting down working as well as the stresses of modern living. Our bodies also reflect our emotions. For example, practitioners point out that rounded shoulders can develop as a fear response to an over-critical parent, while being over-anxious can result in the head being thrust forward instead of balancing easily on top of the spine. These muscular postures tend to become fixed, and in themselves they keep going the emotions originally set off by the symptoms.

Lessons in the Alexander technique usually last 30 to 45 minutes, and you are helped to gradually adjust the way you stand, sit and walk. As I have emphasized throughout this book, it takes time for habits to be changed. During the course of treatment tensions are released and the posture becomes more natural, the ribs open up so that you breathe more naturally and deeply and very often back and neck problems are relieved. As the client becomes more self-aware he or she is able to go through daily life with less stress.

The Alexander technique is a way of learning how to use your body naturally – without effort or tension. Despite the gentleness of the technique, it can bring out profound changes not only in the body but also in the mind, partly through the letting go of old tensions and partly through its training in focussing on the present moment. This can result in a new, more flexible way of dealing with our experiences from unhappiness to stress, which can be particularly useful if you're suffering from insomnia as you acquire a more flexible attitude to your daily life with its problems and difficulties. The technique can help you sleep better by creating greater physical and mental harmony.

AROMATHERAPY

Aromatherapy consists of massage using essential plant oils in a vegetable oil base, and is excellent for relaxation and for relieving tension and stress-related conditions. The essential oils are distilled from the flowers, leaves or roots of plants with specific curative properties. The properties are taken in through the skin into the bloodstream and into both the body and brain through the membranes at the back of the nose. They can affect the organs and glands within the body and have a direct effect on mood since they reach the parts of the brain controlling the emotions. There are oils that can at the same time calm you, clear your brain and lift depression, as well as healing your physical body.

Until recently aromatherapy has been associated mostly with beauty treatments. However, when practised by a qualified aromatherapist, advocates of this treatment claim that it can ease medical conditions such as rheumatic pains. Robert Tisserand pointed out in 1988 that the combination of massage, essential oils and relaxation can boost the immune system and in his book *Aromatherapy for Everyone* gives examples of its therapeutic uses.

A qualified aromatherapist will first make an assessment, usually using a questionnaire, to check on the client's medical history and specific needs, looking in the case of insomnia for its emotional and physical causes before choosing what combination of oils to use. As each oil has several properties you can be treated on several levels at once. The treatment itself can take up to an hour, sometimes longer, and usually the whole body will be massaged. Some find this so relaxing they go to sleep on the massage table while others find that in this relaxed state they can speak about their problems with the therapist. Scents can trigger the emotions and the memory, and clients may find themselves experiencing an emotional release during or after a treatment. As tensions are released, issues come up so that once you're aware of them you're in a better position to be able to deal with them. Your aromatherapist may also suggest nutritional changes or supplements, Bach flower remedies or herbal remedies to take at home.

Aromatherapists may be able to help you come off sleeping pills or tranquillizers, using oils that can both calm you and cleanse your system of the drugs. However, do remember that just as with any other natural therapies it is best to get your doctor's agreement first before starting to come off your sleeping pills.

A full aromatherapy treatment is best given by a professional but your therapist may make up a mixture of oils for you to use at home, perhaps to rub into painful joints or to help you relax in the bath. Oils can also be inhaled, either by putting a drop or two on a handkerchief or by putting a few drops in boiling water and breathing it in. You can buy essential oils in health-food shops and pharmacies, as well as from herbalists. Oils can sometimes be expensive because of the brand name and packaging. Prices can also vary according to the rarity of the plant – for example, blue camomile, which is excellent for insomnia, is expensive.

One of the most helpful oils to promote better sleep is lavender, which is also good for burns, insect bites, period problems and strengthening the immune system. Other oils which are helpful for insomnia are meadowsweet and hops, camomile and orange blossom, marjoram, lemon grass and linden (lime blossom). Geranium helps to create balance and harmony and melissa oil is uplifting and can relieve depression. Any of these oils can be used in the bath.

To aid better sleep, some people find it helpful to put a few drops of an essential oil on the pillow or on a handkerchief before going to bed. You can also smell it if you wake in the night. Lavender is especially good used in this way. You should use only up to four to six drops of oil or oils altogether, using a smaller amount if your skin is very sensitive. If you're using oils at bathtime, stir the water around so the oil spreads evenly and reaches your whole body. Allow yourself time to soak, relax and absorb the oil both through your skin and also by breathing in the vapour. Once oils are mixed they won't retain their properties for very long so they should be kept in a dark air-tight bottle and used within three months. Aromatherapists recommend that the same oil or oil mixture shouldn't be used consecutively for too long as it may lose its effectiveness.

If you have a partner or friend who will give your neck, shoulders and spine a gentle massage, this can help you relax and sleep better. Remember, you should never take aromatherapy oils internally.

BACH FLOWER REMEDIES

The Bach flower remedies were discovered by Dr Edward Bach, a medical doctor who spent his working life seeking ever purer methods of healing. He came to the conclusion that illnesses are caused by negative mental states which, if prolonged, damage physical health. Conversely, happiness, based on being in touch with one's higher self and life's purposes, allows the body to return to its natural state of good health.

In 1934 Dr Bach left his Harley Street practice for the country to try and find plants that were appropriate to specific mental states. By holding his hand over plants to sense their energy he intuitively discovered 38 remedies for different states of mind, testing them on himself and others. He listed seven moods – fear, uncertainty, lack of interest in the present, loneliness, over-sensitivity to influences, despair and over-concern for others. He then subdivided these, finding, for example, seven remedies for different kinds of fear including Mimulus for fear of known causes and Aspen for fear of the unknown. He also created a thirty-ninth, Rescue Remedy, composed of five remedies, to be used for physical and mental shock, accidents and traumas.

To this day the remedies are still prepared according to the method he discovered. Summer flowers and tree blossoms are picked at their best and the heads are floated in a bowl of spring water in full sunlight. According to practitioners of the remedies, after three hours the water starts to bubble and sparkle, filled with the energy of the flowers. The liquid is then strained and poured into a bottle with a small amount of brandy as a preservative. Known as the 'stock' remedy, this reaches the public in small brown bottles with dropper tops. Before they are taken they should be diluted even further so that two drops are added to a small bottle of water. People are usually recommended to take from this four drops four times a day.

Bach remedies can be effective by themselves, or can be used together with other natural treatments. Some practitioners find it more effective to prescribe them one at a time, although up to six remedies can be combined. The length of treatment is highly variable. Sometimes results can be immediate or they may take up to a few months to have an effect. Sometimes the changes they bring about happen so naturally that people only notice the change in themselves when they look back much later.

Advocates of the Bach flower remedies point out that because of their healing effect on our emotional well-being, the remedies can be very helpful with insomnia. Because the remedies are selected according to the individual characteristics, symptoms and attitudes of the person suffering from insomnia, different remedies will suit different people. For example, if your insomnia is caused by a sudden bereavement, suitable remedies might include Star of Bethlehem for shock and Honeysuckle for a tendency to live in the past. Willow is good for resentment, Holly for anger and Olive for exhaustion of mind and body. Oak is a remedy often prescribed for over-conscientiousness. Bach remedies can also help people coming off tranquillizers and sleeping pills by helping them deal better with any old anxieties and worries that can come to the surface during the withdrawal period.

Anyone can treat themselves with the Bach flower remedies with the help of Dr Bach's booklet *The Twelve Healers and Other Remedies*. The remedies can be bought at many health-food shops and pharmacies and some homeopathic pharmacies. As it can be difficult to see oneself clearly enough to decide which remedies are best to take, it may initially be helpful to get advice from an expert practitioner. As you become familiar with the remedies, it becomes easier to select the best remedy for yourself.

HOMEOPATHY

Developed in the 18th century by a German doctor, Samuel Hahnemann, homeopathy is another complete system of medicine which can treat insomniacs on many levels, including the body, mind and energy system. It is based on giving minute doses of natural substances (plants, etc.) which, instead of suppressing symptoms, encourage the body to fight back.

A number of medically trained doctors have taken further training in homeopathy and there and are a few homeopathic hospitals where you can be treated. There are also numbers of homeopathic practitioners who, although they haven't gone through medical school, have usually taken a longer training in homeopathy than qualified doctors.

From a homeopathic viewpoint insomnia isn't something that can be treated in isolation – you have to look at the whole person. Insomnia is often part of a wider pattern related to the way we experience and cope with our daytime anxieties and feelings, which can sometimes go back to patterns developed in childhood or adolescence or result from some later trauma. At the first appointment the practitioner will usually ask the patient a range of questions about his or her emotions, tastes in food, dreams, feelings and attitudes and lifestyle, as well as about any physical symptoms. The remedy or remedies will only be prescribed when a complete picture of the person has been built up, and will be chosen to deal both with the symptoms associated with insomnia and its underlying causes.

Although there are some homeopathic sleeping pills on the market they may not be suitable for everyone. The *Materia Medica*, the basic homeopathic reference book, describes a vast range of types of insomnia such as racing thoughts, early waking, fear, anxiety and feeling worse in the morning, and outlines specific remedies for each. As such, it isn't possible to recommend a blanket remedy for insomnia that would suit everyone. Also, since homeopathic remedies take time to have an effect, there are some risks in trying to treat yourself long term. A homeopathic pharmacist may be willing to make up a remedy for you, but would probably advise you to consult a professional homeopath as well. However, if you're interested in using homeopathy for first aid at home there are many good books available. (*See* 'Further Reading').

For people coming off sleeping pills or other tranquillizers, homeopathic remedies claim to help to strengthen the system at the same time as clearing it. If during withdrawal people find themselves re-experiencing the emotional problems that caused them to become addicted in the first place, a good homeopath will also supply reassurance and counselling or refer patients on for counselling if necessary.

MASSAGE

One of the most ancient and most natural forms of therapy, massage was practised in ancient times in the East, and later by the physicians of Ancient Greece who included it as part of their medical treatment. It has become increasingly popular in the West in the last decade or so and is regarded as a useful therapy by both natural practitioners and hospital nurses. Traditionally the 'healing touch' has long been recognized as therapeutic. Touch and relaxation are healing in themselves.

Massage is another helpful and enjoyable way of dealing with the tensions and stress associated with insomnia. It is especially helpful for people who find it difficult to relax. Lying on the couch, having your body massaged, can ease away all kinds of muscular and mental tensions. Also massage stimulates the circulation of blood and lymph, boosting the flow of oxygen and essential nutrients in the blood, and also helps the body to free itself of waste toxins. This can be particularly beneficial for problems like rheumatism and arthritis.

There are various methods of massage. Probably the best known is Swedish massage, which uses a variety of techniques to relieve stress, encourage circulation, take the tension out of tight muscles and break down fat. A professional massage can take an hour or longer and is a very pleasant experience. These days massage therapists often use aromatherapy oils in their massage oils.

Almost everyone can benefit from massage, from the very young to the very old. The excellent work of Dr Anne Kubler-Ross with people with terminal illnesses shows how the gentle touch of massage can comfort and soothe. She also highlights how older people can benefit greatly from touch and are often starved of it.

Many people find that giving a massage can be as soothing as receiving one. Anyone can give a massage. If you do so, a good idea is to concentrate on the neck and shoulders which are often particular areas of tension. If you are untrained, remember to keep your touch gentle. You can learn a great deal from books such as Lucinda Lidell's *The Book of Massage*, which gives instructions for massage, shiatsu and reflexology with sections on massaging babies and old people as well as explaining energy systems and centres.

Massaging the feet also can be very soothing, mentally and physically. Among other benefits it can draw tension away from the head, helping to calm an over-active mind. Foot massage is an excellent way of helping you drift off to sleep. Trying to give yourself a massage is not as good as someone doing it for you, but it can still be soothing. Starting with your head, try massaging your neck and shoulders, gently pressing and releasing with your palms and fingers. Simply massaging your hands and fingers can also release tension.

MEDICAL HERBALISM

Herbal medicine has been used throughout the ages all over the world and is growing in popularity today in response to concern about drugs and the growing demand by people for more natural forms of medication. Herbalists tend not just to treat symptoms but rather they recommend herbal preparations and medicines aimed at improving general vitality and emotional well-being, clearing the system of toxins and restoring balance and harmony. In this way, medical herbalists claim good sleep then follows naturally. Although herbalism is generally safe and doesn't have the side-effects of pharmaceutical products, herbs are potent substances and you should go to someone who has been properly trained.

As well as assessing symptoms, practitioners evaluate the overall balance of the body's various systems to see if there are any underlying disharmonies. In the treatment of insomnia, the herbalist would want to find out what is contributing to the lack of sleep and will look into the patient's lifestyle, including exercise and nutrition. Herbal medicine can act quite quickly, especially when patients pay attention to a good diet. With chronic or long-standing problems, however, it can take time to restore health as the medicines work gently and thoroughly, both detoxifying the patient's system and building up his or her strength. Treatment is regarded as a joint effort in which patients play their part by making any changes that are recommended to them. Herbalists, like many other natural practitioners, feel that relying on herbs simply as tranquillizers is much the same as relying on medical drugs in that it can lead to a psychological dependence and that you should also deal with the causes of your insomnia.

Herbal drinks

Herb teas are becoming increasingly popular as replacements for caffeine-containing drinks. There is a wide variety of herbal teabags in the shops, some of them specially blended to help you relax or sleep. As they can be quite expensive, you may choose to buy loose herbs from a herbalist or health-food shop and try out single herbs or your own mixture of herbs. Herbs can lose their efficacy over time so it's a good idea to buy them in small quantities and keep them in an air-tight jar, using them fairly quickly.

Herbal infusions are slightly stronger than teas and herbal practitioners recommend that they can be taken medicinally up to three times a day. You can make up your own infusion of one or more herbs, using 1–2 heaped teaspoonfuls of dried leaves or flowers per cup. Use a small teapot and pour the water onto the herbs when the water is just on the boil. Then leave the liquid to stand, covered, for at least five to ten minutes before drinking it.

Herbs that help sleep include camomile, which is one of the best-known herbs for calming the nerves and for settling the digestion. It is said to have cumulative effects, becoming more effective over a period of time. Some people find the flavour bland and it has the disadvantage of being mildly diuretic. Lime flower (linden) makes a pleasantly flavoured and effective nightcap and is good for headaches, nervous tension and general restlessness. *Scutellaria laterifolia* (skullcap) is a tonic as well as a sedative. It is high in magnesium and calcium which help to strengthen the nervous system. *Passiflora* (passion-flower) has also got a good reputation for helping to restore good sleep and is an ingredient of many herbal sleeping pills. Valerian root is well known as a sedative. However, it has an unpleasant smell and taste and so most people find it best mixed with more pleasant-flavoured herbs. It has a stronger effect than many herbs and some people find it gives them headaches when they drink it in large amounts.

Herbs can also by used in the bath by making an extra-strong mixture or infusion, steeped, strained and poured into your bath water. Lime flowers and hops are helpful for insomnia. Make an infusion by pouring a cup of boiling water over a bowl containing three crushed heads of lime flowers and keep this covered for ten minutes. You can also use lavender or a mixture of herbs. You can also try filling a muslin bag with the heads and tying it to the hot tap so that the hot water runs through it. Before getting into the bath, add a strained infusion of the same herbs.

If you take a herbal remedy for a chronic or long-standing condition, practitioners claim that you can expect some improvement within two or three days, but it may take two or more weeks to get the full effect. When you do improve, taper off gradually. Herbs are not truly addictive in a physical sense but they may lead to reliance on them and psychological dependency. Also, practitioners point out that as they act upon the central nervous system they shouldn't be taken regularly for weeks on end.

NATUROPATHY

Naturopathy, which is also sometimes called nature cure, is one of the oldest and best-established forms of natural and holistic medicine. It's based on the principle that the body has its own restorative and curative powers and so under the right conditions will heal itself. The right conditions for good health include nutrition, exercise, relaxation, a balanced and unstressed muscular–skeletal system and a positive outlook on life. Treatment consists mainly in trying to remove the obstacles to health rather than adding extra forms of cures. However, many naturopaths use some herbal and homeopathic preparations as well as nutritional supplements according to their assessment of the client's needs. Many naturopaths are also trained in osteopathy which helps to relieve structural and muscular tensions and pain.

Some practitioners may advocate fasting so that the body can get rid of accumulated toxins – either a complete fast or a few days of fruit or fruit juices. Fasting doesn't suit everyone, and the naturopath will take your personal needs and system into account before recommending it. Naturopaths not only advise on nutrition but also look at your whole lifestyle, including your working life and any anxieties causing particular stresses. They will also advise on appropriate exercise and relaxation techniques and support you in making changes to your lifestyle. Their approach to the treatment of insomnia is based on addressing the underlying problems.

OSTEOPATHY AND CHIROPRACTIC

These two methods of treating the bones, muscles and joints that make up our muscular–skeletal system are becoming increasingly accepted by orthodox medicine.

Developed independently of each other in the US towards the end of the 19th century, the two methods have differences although some techniques are used by both. There are also differences in the techniques used by practitioners from different training schools.

Both osteopathy and chiropractic are based on the principle that the health of the spine has a profound effect on overall well-being. An extension of the brain, the spinal cord connects with all the organs of the body by means of the circulatory and nervous systems. So although people generally seek these therapies for back and joint pain they can be helpful for a wide range of problems – for example, asthma, migraine, indigestion and pre-menstrual tension. Some practitioners, particularly those who have also trained in naturopathy, take a particular interest in nutrition and can advise you on diet and supplements.

Manipulating and adjusting the spinal vertebrae isn't usually painful, and the effects can be extremely relaxing. Neck pains, for example, can often lead to insomnia and chiropractic treatment can relieve the pain and help restore a good sleep pattern. Practitioners report that more and more elderly people are turning to these therapies for help with arthritic and back pain with good results. Manipulation may not cure arthritis but it can relieve the pressure on arthritic joints and improve the circulation of blood around them. Practitioners use a variety of techniques as well as direct manipulation. These include soft-tissue techniques, which are specific ways of massaging the muscles, as well as methods that can help to realign joints, relax over-tense bodies and encourage good blood circulation.

Manipulative techniques can often help insomniacs and not just by relieving pain in the back or other joints.

Treatment can be an excellent stress-reliever. For example, insomnia, headaches, migraines and general tension are often linked to problems in the neck vertebrae, which both the osteopath and the chiropractor can relieve or cure.

REFLEXOLOGY

Records exist which show that reflexology techniques were practised by the ancient Egyptians. Reflexology was rediscovered in the 1920s by an American physician, Dr William Fitzgerald, and is becoming increasingly popular as a form of natural therapy.

As well as being a natural therapeutic treatment for a number of ailments, reflexology is also deeply relaxing. Practitioners point out that quite often clients drop off to sleep while their feet are being manipulated. Like acupuncture, it is based on the theory that channels of energy flow through the body, although these energy channels are not the same in both therapies. In the case of reflexology, there are ten channels which can be tapped into through specific reflex zones in the feet and hands. The feet themselves represent a kind of map of the body with the big toes relating to the head and neck and the bony side of the foot to the spine. Reflex points for the liver, kidneys and other organs are found in the soft part of the feet.

Reflexologists are trained to find energy blocks in the feet and use massage techniques to unblock them, stimulating the energy flow and encouraging the body to heal itself. Some patients can actually sense the energy in the part of the body relating to the point on the foot being treated. Generally, reflexology is a fairly painless treatment, although sometimes pressure on a specific site of trouble can hurt. However, this doesn't last long. You may be treated sitting up or lying down. The practitioner will give a complete treatment to both feet and then focus on any problem areas.

Practitioners point out that reflexology is very good for the relief of a whole range of problems, such as chronic pain, hormonal imbalances and a variety of other problems that may be affecting your sleep. The therapy is also good for releasing stress, tension and emotional build-up so that good sleep can follow. For insomnia, specific attention is usually given to parts of the foot which reflect problems in the head area including the pituitary gland – the master gland of the hormonal system – and to the adrenals which may be overworked by stress. The solar plexus, which is about a third of the way down the sole of the foot, is another point that is likely to receive attention, and you may be asked to breathe deeply while it is being treated. After a reflexology treatment most people sleep extra well. As with other natural therapies, a course of several treatments will usually be needed to bring about a long-term effect.

SHIATSU

Shiatsu is a form of oriental massage developed in Japan at the beginning of the 20th century. It's based on the same principles as acupuncture but uses the hands, fingers, knuckles and even elbows to stimulate the acupuncture points and rebalance the meridians. Like acupuncture, shiatsu aims to rebalance the body's energy system and so relieve aches and pains, tension and stress. A shiatsu practitioner may show you how to self-massage the points that will help you relax and improve your sleep.

SPIRITUAL HEALING

This form of healing is numerically the largest of the natural therapies, and is becoming increasingly popular as a growing number of people recognize that human beings consist of more than just the material, physical body. Some people are wary of spiritual healing because it can't be fully explained and because of its spiritualist associations. However, there should be nothing weird about a healing session. Healers hold a variety of beliefs and belong to all kinds of religious denominations, or to none at all. And while many healers and spiritualists regard their gifts as being helped by spirit helpers, this is by no means always the case. These days, the power of healing is often explained in terms of the body's energy system rather than in terms of spirits or the spirit world as such.

The common theme in most forms of spiritual healing is the belief in a cosmic or divine energy which is totally benign and loving. Healers see themselves as channels for this energy which is transferred to patients through the healer's hands – or by the healer's thoughts in the case of distant healing. Imbalances caused by emotional trauma and physical stress appear within the energy field before they appear as bodily symptoms. Usually it's in the energy field that healing starts. Through the transference of healing energy, healers claim that harmony is restored to mind, body and spirit – hence the term 'spiritual healing'.

A healing session can last from about 20 minutes to an hour or so. The healer will usually speak with you first and then ask you to sit or lie down. Many of them work almost entirely with the energy field where they claim that they can sense problem areas around the body. Others will lay their hands directly on painful areas, often relieving pain very quickly. Many combine the two techniques. Healing is usually a very relaxing experience and practitioners point out that its calming and uplifting effects on mind and body can be extremely helpful with insomnia. Some people go to sleep during the healing session while others report that they sleep especially well afterwards. Patients often leave a session feeling emotionally and spiritually uplifted. Healers can also provide regular support for people going through difficult times, help them express pent-up emotions and encourage them to build up their own inner resources.

As with any other sort of natural therapy, results are rarely instant. The time it will take to bring about improvement depends very much on the condition and characteristics of the individual patient, as well as on other factors such as how long they have had their problem. Although faith isn't necessary, practitioners point out that patients can aid the healing process by being open-minded. Some people report that they feel the energy flowing from the healer as a hot or cold current or a pleasant tingling. It isn't necessary to feel anything, however, for healing to take place.

Many healers claim clairvoyant or strongly intuitive gifts which can help them to pinpoint the causes of people's problems. Some healers are also good intuitive counsellors, and healer training courses increasingly emphasize the development of counselling skills. It is important, they say, to heal not only the physical but the emotional and spiritual causes of illness. A number of them encourage patients to take part in the release of past stresses through such methods as visualization, meditation and forgiveness.

Conclusion

We began this book by looking at how and why we need sleep and the nature and consequences of insomnia. Now that you have accurate information about sleep you are in a better position to deal with your problem and not add to your worries by unnecessarily worrying about sleep itself. We then looked at the causes of insomnia. If you suffer from insomnia the first thing you need to know is the nature of the problem. Now that you have learned about the nature of sleep and insomnia and how to assess yourself to find out how much sleep you actually get, you're in a position to know the nature of your sleep problem.

Self-monitoring and diary-keeping allow us to know the exact nature of the problem – how much and when you sleep at night as well as the way you go about your daily life. You will probably have been surprised at some mistaken beliefs that you may have had.

We also looked at the various strategies, techniques and therapies that can help promote better sleep. Make a note of the ones that are suitable for your own problem and then make your own treatment plan. Remember, everybody's sleep needs are different and most of us from time to time experience the odd sleepless night. Worrying about not sleeping will only make the problem worse.

Once you've made the decision to tackle insomnia you may recognize that you will have to make changes in the rest of your life. We have seen how insomnia is often a reflection of difficulties in our daily lives – our lifestyle may be too slow or too fast or we may be troubled by our moods and emotions. This book shows us ways to look at our usual methods of coping. It shows us how to identify our beliefs and the way they influence what we think about ourselves and other people and how to challenge those beliefs that are no longer helpful to us.

As we have seen, there are many ways of bringing about change, such as by aiming towards a more balanced lifestyle, through using relaxation and meditation techniques and by learning better ways of coping with our emotions. Some of you may wish to explore the natural therapies. Whatever the methods you choose, remember that anything newly learned needs time and practice to become established. Old patterns of thinking and behaving have taken us time – sometimes a lifetime – to develop so it's not surprising that new ways take time and practice. The important thing to remember is to stick with it. From time to time you may slip into the old habits. Don't despair and give up or think none of your efforts have been worthwhile. Simply go back to the basic principles you have learned that have helped you overcome insomnia, give yourself a quick revision course and with some practice pretty soon you'll be back on track.

Further Reading

Bach, Dr Edward, *The Twelve Healers and Other Remedies*, C. W. Daniel, Saffron Walden, 1989

Boericka, William, *The Homeopathic Materia Medica with Repertory*, The Homeopathic Bookservice, Sittingbourne, 1987

Clover, Dr Anne, *Homeopathy: A Patient's Guide*, Thorsons, Wellingborough, 1984

Courtney, Anthea, *Natural Sleep*, Thorsons, Wellingborough, 1990

Cummings, Stephen and Dana Ullman, *Everybody's Guide to Homeopathic Medicines*, Gollancz, London, 1989

Douglas, Jo and Naomi Richman, *My Child Won't Sleep*, Penguin Books, London, 1984

Fanning, Patrick, *Visualization for Change*, New Harbinger Publications, Oakland, CA, 1994

Graham, Helen, *A Picture of Health*, Piatkus, London, 1995

Harvey, David, *The Power of Healing*, Aquarian Press, London, 1983

Horne, James, *Why We Sleep*, Oxford University Press, Oxford, 1988

Lambley, Peter, *Insomnia and Other Sleeping Problems*, Sphere, 1982

Lidell, Lucinda, *The Book of Massage*, Ebury Press, London, 1984

McCormick, Elizabeth, *Change for the Better*, Unwin, London, 1990

Shakti, Gawain, *Creative Visualization*, Whatever Publishing, Mill Valley, CA, 1978

—— *The Creative Visualization Workbook*, New World Library, Berkeley, CA, 1992

Tisserand, Robert, *Aromatherapy for Everyone*, Penguin Books, London, 1988

Further Help

Should your insomnia continue despite your efforts you many need additional help. The first step is to discuss your problem with your family doctor who may recommend that you seek specialist help and refer you to a clinical psychologist or to a sleep clinic near to where you live.

Countries differ in how people can best get further help. In the US for example, you may contact the American Sleep Disorders Association directly and receive their list of contacts in your area. In the UK it is best to contact your family doctor as the British Sleep Society only distributes its contact numbers to health-care professionals.

If you live too far away from a sleep disorder centre to attend appointments, telephone the centre nearest you as they may know of someone in your area who can help.

Australia

Australasian Sleep Association (ASA)
President Ron Grunstein MD
Sleep Disorders Centre
Royal Prince Alfred Hospital
Missenden Road
Camperdown
NSW 2050
Tel: 612 9515 8630
Fax: 612 9365 5612

Canada

Clarke Institute of Psychiatry
250 College Street
Toronto 2B

Ontario
Tel: (416) 979-2221

Sleep Laboratories
Dept of Medicine
Ottawa General Hospital
Ottawa
Ontario KIN 4C8
Tel: (613) 231–4738

UK

The British Sleep Society aims to promote the study and treatment of sleep disorders but does not offer a direct service to the public.

The Directory of Chartered Psychologists – via public libraries or from the British Psychological Society, St Andrews House, 48 Princess Road East, Leicester LE1 7DR. Tel: 0116 254 9568.

Self-Help
Sleep Trust: Tel: 01635 44593
Tel: Sleep Matters Tel: 0181 994 9874

USA

American Sleep Disorders Association
6301 Bandel Road
Suite 101
Rochester
MN 55901
Tel: (507) 287 6006
Fax: (507) 287 6008

The staff at the ASDA Nation Office is available Monday to Friday, 8am to 5pm CST. They will answer your questions and assist you. For further information, you may contact them on 507 287 6006.

Useful Addresses

ACUPUNCTURE

Australia

Acupuncture Ethics and
    Standards Organization
PO Box 84
Merrylands
NSW
Tel: 296 827882

Canada

Acupuncture Foundation of
    Canada
7321 Victoria Park Avenue
Unit 18
Markham
Ontario L3R 2Z3
Tel: 905 881 5540

New Zealand

NZRA
P O Box 9950
Wellington 1
Tel: 00648 016 400

South Africa

Western Cape Su Jok
    Acupuncture
    Institute
3 Periwinkle Close
Kommetjie 7975
Tel: 021 783 3460

UK

British Acupuncture
    Council (BAC)
Park House
206–208 Latimer Road
London W10 6RE
Tel: 0181 964 0222

USA

American Association
    of Acupuncture
    and Oriental
    Medicine
1424 16th Street NW
Suite 501
Washington DC 20036

AROMATHERAPY

Australia

International Federation of
   Aromatherapists
1/390 Burwood Road
Hawthorn
BIC 3122, Australia
Tel: 03 9530 0067

South Africa

Association of
   Aromatherapists
PO Box 23924
Claremont 7735
Tel: 021 531 297

UK

Aromatherapy Trades Council
3 Latymer Close
Braybrooke
Market Harborough
Leicester LE16 8LN
Tel: 01858 465 731

International Federation of
   Aromatherapists
Stamford House
Chiswick High Road
London W4 1TH
Tel: 0181 742 2605

International Society of
   Professional
   Aromatherapists

82 Ashby Road
Hinckley
Leicestershire LE10 1AG
Tel: 01455 637 987

USA

American Alliance of
   Aromatherapy
PO Box 750428
Petaluma
California 94975-0428

American Aromatherapy
   Association
PO Box 3679
South Pasadena
California 91031

National Association of
   Holistic Aromatherapy
PO Box 17622
Boulder
Colorado 80308-0622

COUNSELLING AND
PSYCHOTHERAPY

UK

British Association for
   Counselling
1 Regent Place
Rugby
Warwicks CV21 2PJ
Tel: 01788 550899/578328
Fax: 01788 562189

British Association of
  Psychotherapists
37 Mapesbury Road
London NW2 4HJ
Tel: 0181 452 9823
Fax: 0181 452 5182

The Institute of Stress
  Management
57 Hall Lane
London NW4 4TJ

UK Council for Psychotherapy
167–9 Great Portland Street
London W1N 5F
Tel: 0171 436 3002
Fax: 0171 436 3013

USA

American Counseling
  Association
5999 Stevenson Avenue
Alexandrea
Virginia 22304-9800

American Psychological
  Association
750 First Street NE
Washington
DC 20002
Tel: 415 327 2066

HERBALISM

Australia

National Herbalists
  Association of Australia

Suite 305, BST House
3 Small Street
Broadway, NSW 2007
Tel: 02 211 6437

Canada

Canadian Natural Health
  Association
439 Wellington Street
Toronto
Ontario M5V 2H7
Tel: 416 977 2642

South Africa

South African Naturopaths
  and Herbalists Association
PO Box 18663
Wynberg 7824

UK

The General Council and
  Register of Consultant
  Herbalists
Grosvenor House
49 Seaway
Middleton-on-Sea
Sussex PO22 7SA
Tel: 01243 586012

National Institute of
  Medical Herbalists
56 Longbrooke Street
Exeter EX4 8HA
Tel: 01392 426 022

School of Herbal Medicine/
    Phytotherapy
Bucksteep Manor
Bodle Street Green
Near Hailsham
Sussex BN27 4RJ

USA

American Herbalists
    Guild
PO Box 1683
Sequel
California 95073
Tel: 408 484 2441

HOMEOPATHY

Australia

Australian Federation of
    Homeopaths
238 Ballarat Road
Footscray
Victoria 3011
Tel: 03 9318 3057

Canada

Canadian Society of
    Homeopathy
87 Meadowlands Drive
    West
Nepean
Ontario K2G 2R9

New Zealand

New Zealand Homeopathic
    Society
Box 2299
Auckland
Tel: 9 630 9458

UK

British Homoepathic
    Association
27a Devonshire Street
London W1N 1RJ
Tel/Fax: 0171 935 2163

USA

American Institute of
    Homeopathy
1585 Glencoe
Denver CO 80220
Tel: 303 370 9164

International Foundation for
    Homeopathy
2366 Eastlake Avenue
East Suit 301
Seattle WA 98102
Tel: 206 776 4147

National Center for
    Homeopathy
801 North Fairfax Street
Alexandria
Virginia 22314
Tel: 703 548 7790

Index